HOW THE
LIGHT SHINES

"Using her lived experience and thorough research, Trisha Elliott provides practical suggestions to ground oneself spiritually as caregiver. How The Light Shines is an encouraging book for caregivers and for those supporting them."
– Rev. Lynn McGrath, Minister at Agassiz United Church, Agassiz, BC

"This important book by Trisha Elliott encourages us to look at the caregiving role as a 'sacred call' that can act as a potential gateway into a deeper relationship with ourselves, our loved ones and the spiritual realm. The central premise is that caregivers have a higher purpose, and that the divine can be found in the most mundane and most challenging work. By focusing on the inner and outer resources available to caregivers and the restorative potential of creative expression, this book is a positive, practical guide to finding meaning, support and healing in troubled times. Like light shining through a stained glass window, these uplifting ideas, references and exercises have the potential to restore our souls by transforming the mundane into the holy."
– Chris White, Musician and Community Developer, Ottawa, Canada

HOW THE LIGHT SHINES

STORIES, STRATEGIES, AND SPIRITUAL PRACTICES FOR CAREGIVERS OF PEOPLE WITH DEMENTIA

TRISHA ELLIOTT

WOOD LAKE

Editor: Mike Schwartzentruber
Proofreader: Dianne Greenslade
Designer: Robert MacDonald
Author photographer: Isaac Elliott-Perreault

Library and Archives Canada Cataloguing in Publication
Title: How the light shines : stories, strategies, and spiritual practices for caregivers of
people with dementia / Trisha Elliott.
Names: Elliott, Trisha, author.
Description: [New edition] | Previously published: Kelowna, BC : Wood Lake, 2021.
Includes bibliographical references.
Identifiers: Canadiana 20210354305 | ISBN 9781773435268 (softcover)
Subjects: LCSH: Caregivers – Religious life. | LCSH: Dementia – Patients – Care. |
LCSH: Dementia – Religious aspects – Christianity. | LCSH: Christian life.
Classification: LCC BV4910.9 .E45 2021 | DDC 259/.4196831 – dc23

ISBN 978-1-77343-526-8

Published by Wood Lake Publishing Inc.
485 Beaver Lake Road, Kelowna, BC, Canada V4V 1S5
www.woodlake.com | 250.766.2778

Wood Lake Publishing acknowledges the financial support of
the Government of Canada. Wood Lake Publishing acknowledges the financial support
of the Province of British Columbia through the Book Publishing Tax Credit.

Wood Lake Publishing acknowledges that we operate in the unceded territory of
the Syilx/Okanagan People, and we work to support reconciliation and challenge the
legacies of colonialism. The Syilx/Okanagan territory is a diverse and beautiful
landscape of deserts and lakes, alpine forests and endangered grasslands.
We honour the ancestral stewardship of the Syilx/Okanagan People.

Printed in Canada
Printing 10 9 8 7 6 5 4 3 2 1

CONTENTS

For Patricia and Floyd Elliott
and Donelda and Clifford Irving
who taught me what it means to care.

**The light shines in the darkness,
and the darkness did not overcome it.**
John 1:1–5

PREFACE

For over two decades, I've been caring for both caregivers and people with dementia in my role as a church minister. During that time, what has struck me most is that while caregivers I've supported often describe the heavy tasks and dilemmas associated with caring, few consider their care itself as sacred, holy work.

I believe we are nearest to God when we do what God does most – love and care. As such, caregivers are closest to the heart of God. Applying that lens to caregiving can change the experience, making difficult times more bearable and joyful times more apparent. That's why I've written this book for caregivers of persons with dementia who have a desire not only to hone their caring skills, but also to deepen their relationship with God through their care. This book explores feelings of loss and challenge, but turns toward potential and hope.

Each chapter explores a dimension of the caregiving experience. The themes are inspired by topics and issues caregivers have raised with me over the years. Each chapter applies a fresh, caregiving lens to a beloved Bible story; pivots around personal experiences of caregiving; contains information, tips, or advice from experts in the field; and is followed by questions for reflection or discussion for individuals and groups, a spiritual practice, and a prayer.

Many people have contributed to this work. The strategies and insights come from decades of experience caring for people with dementia and their caregivers, as well as from colleagues and seminars, personal study, and hands-on experience. I am deeply indebted to all my teachers over the years; this book represents the best I've learned from them.

Some of my loved ones have dementia. For a variety of reasons, they are uncomfortable with sharing their diagnosis. Naming my experience would mean naming theirs. While I am not sharing my personal experiences in this book out of respect for my loved ones, they very much inform my approach and perspectives.

I have changed the names of those whose experiences I describe in this book, as well as any identifying details where I have not been able to gain consent because the persons quoted or implicated in the quotes can no longer give it. Though these details may have been changed, the scenarios and quotes are real. I am deeply grateful for those who shared their experiences with me in the course of writing this book.

Language has limitations. Some prefer to refer to dementia as an illness, others a disability. These are important ways of framing the reality of dementia. Throughout this book I refer to dementia as a "condition."

Similarly, there is considerable conversation in circles of support about whether caregivers should be called carers, care partners, or some other term. It's really up to us as individuals and to those we are in a caring relationship with to name and define our roles. I've used the term "caregiver" because I believe it's more generally recognizable, but I hope that those who prefer to use other terms are able to identify just as well.

Along those same lines, there isn't only one kind of caregiver. The time we commit to caregiving, the type of tasks and responsibilities our caring entails, the geographic region in which we care, the supports we have available, our relationship with the one we are caring for, and so many other variables mean that caregivers are a diverse group. I've tried to share a range of scenarios in this book, and I hope that caregivers of all stripes will identify with them.

Most importantly, caregiving is often a two-way street. Although this book is for caregivers and focuses on the practice of caregiving, I have included exchanges with persons who have dementia and every chapter begins with their voice. I strongly believe that all of our caring should take its lead from the person we are caring for.

1
Responding to God's Call

"I know I'm going to have to go on.
Am I making sense? Sometimes I don't. I get mixed up.
God knows, though. I know God cares."

– Joy

Caregiving is typically understood as an activity, as what we do. Likely, because we caregivers do a lot. But caregiving is deeper than what we *do*. It is more than a series of tasks.

It is, first, a call to love.

Have you ever thought about caregiving as a sacred call? As *your* sacred call?

When the biblical authors wanted to describe caregiving, they told stories of shepherding. In ancient times, people were well aware of what shepherds did to care for their sheep. Even today, caregiving is so synonymous with shepherding that congregations are referred to as flocks and religious leaders as "pastors," which literally means "to lead to pasture." We might not know much about shepherding in the first century, but caregivers know what it's like to have mountainous tasks, to live with uncertainty, and to hang on to precious feelings of contentment. The shepherd's story is one we are familiar with.

Shepherding was an effort to keep the flock together and safe. The shepherd scanned the rocky terrain for holes, poking them with his staff to scare out scorpions and snakes, his nail-studded rod at the ready to fend off jackals and hyenas. Some days, counting and keeping track of all the coming and going seemed endless; nights guarding the open sheepfolds tiresome. The worry could be relentless: What if I can't find pasture, or I run out of food during the winter? What if the current in the stream spooks the sheep?

But there were other moments, too. Ones that the shepherd wouldn't trade: the elation of the shearing festival; gentle moments playing the flute under a starry, silent night; the intimacy of slathering the sheeps' wounds with olive oil; the connection that deepened each time the shepherd called the sheep by name and their woolly heads crooked at the slightest sound of his voice; the satisfaction of bringing them home when they'd been swept down a stream or had wandered off.

"Feed my sheep," Jesus told Peter, one of his disciples. In other words, care like a shepherd.

Just as caring is the vocation of the shepherd, so it is to be ours. The word vocation comes from the Latin *vocare*, meaning "to call" or "voice." In Christian terms, a vocation refers to a call from God, usually to some form of service.

Minister types like me aren't the only ones who have vocations. Jesus called ordinary people such as business owners and general labourers who were going about their ordinary lives to follow him. The vast majority of the time, God's call wasn't to leave their work, it was to heed

God's voice within the work they were already doing.

The idea of finding God in work is summed up beautifully in a single Hebrew word: *avodah*. *Avodah* is used to reference working and worshipping.[1] In other words, work isn't something we do all week and worship isn't just what happens on Sunday. The idea behind the word *avodah* is that work can be a place of intimate connection with God. Worship and work are interconnected.

The care you offer is a special, meaningful, sacred call. It is *avodah*. It's work and it's deeply spiritual. It is a vocation.

What would change for you if you saw your work as sacred – if you saw each and every task as an extension of God's grace?

"You've got to be joking," I said, brushing off my colleague when she told me that cleaning the house was a spiritual practice for her. For me, it's usually just one more thing at the end of a long week that I don't have time or energy for. A necessary evil.

"Change how you look at it," she advised. "Focus on the task at hand, not on the giant to-do list, and ask God to meet you in the work."

I agreed, albeit with great skepticism. I put on some uplifting tunes and got busy dusting my baseboards, talking to God all the while. Surprisingly, shifting my approach changed the experience. Now, scrubbing the floors has become a sacred time to connect with God.

I'm not trying to convince you to like cleaning or any other task on your to-do list. What I *am* saying is that God can be found even in the most mundane work. And frankly, caregiving can involve a lot of boring, repetitive, and even repulsive tasks. Yet even and perhaps especially in the basic things we do, caregivers have a higher purpose.

Jesus spent most of his time either giving care himself, or calling people to the work of caregiving. He saw the best in people and was a companion to all who were deemed unworthy. He tended to those who are sick and dying. He paid the ultimate cost for advocating for the marginalized. And he called followers to do the same. Whether they were serving meals to thousands on a hill, supporting vulnerable widows or providing for orphans, followers of Jesus were called, above all things, to "love God and love your neighbour." In other words, to give care. Caregiving is the holy call of Jesus. It is love lived out.

When we give care, we walk on sacred ground. We are invited into people's most vulnerable moments, ones reserved for precious few. There, in the sacred ground of vulnerability, God is most alive. As caregivers, we live out our vocation, our call to care, by being witnesses, companions, healers, and advocates.

In our role as witnesses, we see what others outside the caregiving relationship don't. We have a front row seat to pain, struggle, and sorrow. We are the ones who remain at the foot of the cross, who are present in suffering and who don't run away. We are witnesses like Jesus' mother and his mother's sister, Mary and Mary Magdalene, who stood at the foot of his cross, feeling all the grief, anger, powerlessness, and love, and yet refusing to abandon their loved one.

We can feel at times that witnessing is a burden and surely it can be. It's also a privilege. There are very few people in our lives who will stick with us in pain and with whom we would want to share our deepest aches.

When profound things happen in life, we often rush to tell someone so that they, too, can witness what happened; so that they, too, can share what we feel. But daily challenges don't seem so newsworthy. Getting

14

groceries might be a herculean task, for us, but there are few people we would call to tell. Caregivers are witnesses to daily suffering and triumphs, things that no one would speak of but which matter. Your witness is a blessing, your presence a healing balm, even and especially when your loved one can't tell you so. Don't underestimate what your presence means.

We can't take away pain and suffering, but our companionship makes a difference. When we are alone, our perspective becomes very small; our focus narrows to our own experience. With someone else at our side, we see ourselves through their eyes. Just by being present, caregivers can provide perspective to others and help them see themselves and what they are experiencing in a broader, healing light.

You are a healer. Have you thought about your caring that way? Caregivers are rarely *"curers,"* but we are often healers. There's a difference between healing and curing. We are not going to cure our loved one's dementia. Nothing we can do will take away the condition. But through our commitment to bear witness to the struggle of our loved one and to be a present companion through it, we offer healing. Healing is about making something or someone whole. Caregivers have the capacity to heal hearts, settle minds, and boost spirits. Through our love, we promote wholeness. In promoting wholeness, we observe and act on what diminishes the spirit.

Very often, we stand in our loved one's corner as advocates and as justice seekers. We advocate for quality care in healthcare settings, and for inclusion in our communities, social circles, and networks. We strive to destigmatize dementia. Through our advocacy, we widen the circle of care, transforming not only the life of the person we are caring for, but expanding the loving capacity of all those around us. We may not set out to change the world, but when we strive for better care and for social inclusion, there's a ripple effect.

Years ago, I got a call from Teresa, a caregiver. She wanted to know what my church was doing to include people with dementia because she wanted to find a church to attend with her dad. I stammered around. Honestly, we weren't intentional about it. "Anyone can attend any of our events. We try to include everyone. Please come to anything we are running and we will accommodate," I said.

"But what are you doing to specifically welcome people like my dad who have dementia," Teresa pressed.

I didn't know how to answer. "What should we be doing?" I asked.

She rapidly rhymed off a list. "Make your congregation more accepting so that if my dad wanders or talks during the service, I don't feel bad. Find ways to include him in things that don't require him to remember. You can train volunteers to look out for ways the church can be more inclusive. Get rid of carpets that can slide, paint a neon strip across the stairs so that my dad can see them easier. You know, stuff like that."

No, I didn't know. But I learned. Thanks to Teresa's advocacy for her dad, my leadership ability developed, and my awareness expanded. By simply making a call, she helped us live more deeply into God's vision for a world where all are welcome. Even when we aren't intentional about it, caregivers become agents of social change.

Few of us know the impact we have as witnesses, companions, healers, and advocates. Many of us don't even set out to be caregivers; we are pressed into the role and feel ill-equipped for the job. That's understandable. The Bible is full of characters who didn't want to be called.

The prophet Jeremiah felt he was too young and inexperienced to accept God's call. Moses pleaded with God not to send him to Egypt – among other things, he objected that he wasn't eloquent enough. When God called Jonah, he literally ran away. God went to great lengths to get his attention, laughably holding him captive in the belly of a whale. Most of Jesus' disciples fumbled their way along. They just tried to do their best to get through the day without any major screw-ups. A lot of times, they failed.

Regardless of how you came to give care or how well you feel you are doing it, God is working through you. You don't have to be perfect to love.

There's a brilliant, enormous stained-glass window in one of the churches I served. Each of the heavily soldered panels are textured, the colours so brilliant that when light shines through an abstract image is cast on the adjacent wall. I always marvel at how stained-glass windows, among the church's most prized architectural features, consist of bits of broken glass. There are lessons in their composition: nothing – and no one – is so broken that it, that *we*, can't be made beautiful. On good and bad days, in sickness and in health, we radiate God's light. The unexpected and ever-changing pattern the window casts may be just as or more beautiful than the window itself.

Caregiving is about holding vulnerability to the light of God. A light that always shines, always heals, always comforts and blesses, always conveys beauty.

You are the light God shines through. Don't let your care be diminished. Yours is a sacred call.

Psalm 23, arguably the Bible's most travelled passage, doesn't begin by referring to God in an abstract way, as in "God is a shepherd or like a shepherd." It begins in a deeply personal way: "God is *my* shepherd." God isn't whiling away time on a cloud somewhere, either. God is busy, *leading* us to still waters and righteous paths, *restoring* our soul. Even when we walk through the darkest valleys, God is there, *protecting* us, *preparing* a table before us, *anointing* us, *filling* our cup to overflowing. Thanks to the shepherd's care, goodness and mercy follow us all the days of our life. Not some days. Not just the good days. But *all* the days, even and especially the bad ones.

In your call to care – as you witness, accompany, heal, and advocate – know this: you are never alone. God is shepherding you.

SCRIPTURE: PSALM 23

The Lord is my shepherd,
    I shall not want.
He makes me lie down in
    green pastures;
he leads me beside still
    waters;
he restores my soul.
He leads me in right paths
    for his name's sake.

Even though I walk through the
    darkest valley,
I fear no evil;
    for you are with me;
    your rod and your staff –
    they comfort me.

You prepare a table before me
    in the presence of my
    enemies;
you anoint my head with oil;
    my cup overflows.
Surely goodness and mercy
    shall follow me
all the days of my life,
and I shall dwell in the house of
    the Lord
my whole life long.

QUESTIONS FOR REFLECTION AND DISCUSSION

1. Do you think about caregiving as a holy call? Why or why not? What would change if you did?
2. How did Jesus play the caregiver role of witness, companion, healer, and advocate?

3. When have you played these roles? Which one comes most naturally? Which one doesn't? Are there others?

4. When do you most sense God's presence when you care?

SPIRITUAL PRACTICE: MEDITATIVE VISUALIZATION

Visualization is about imagining potential. When it is used in an intentionally spiritual way, it can help us become more aware of the presence of God and more able to sense God's lead. When we visualize ourselves in scripture, we become acquainted with the spirit of Christ who meets us there.

1. Breathe deeply several times.

2. Feel your muscles relax, imagining the tension leaving your body.

3. Read Psalm 23. Visualize walking around the scenes of the passage. Explore the green pastures, the still waters, the lush valleys, the abundant table, and the loving home.

4. Now visualize yourself caring for your loved one. Imagine your typical day. Where are the green pastures and still waters in your day? Where is God? How is God present to you?

5. Imagine the shadow moments in your caring. How is God present to you? What is God saying?

6. Imagine the right paths, the places on your caregiving journey where you are living out your call to care most gracefully. How is God present to you? What is God saying?

7. Write down the essence of what God said to you in your visualization. Place it in a prominent spot or carry it with you. Let the words guide you.

PRAYER

Holy One, you are my Great Shepherd.

When my call to care wavers, you restore me.

When the path is unclear, you lead me.

When the way is joyful, you are with me.

When my energy wanes, you prepare a table before me.

When the shadows loom, you comfort me.

When my compassion deepens, you anoint me.

When I'm lost, you lead me home.

All the days of my life, O God

you are with me.

My cup overflows with your love.

Amen.

2

Discerning the Still, Small Voice

"I'd like to be treated like a real person.
Like I'm alive."
– John

These are the facts: there are over 100 types of dementia affecting over 50 million people around the world.[2] Most of us equate dementia with Alzheimer's disease, likely because 60 to 80 percent of the time, Alzheimer's is the cause of dementia.[3] But dementia is actually an umbrella term for a number of generally progressive conditions that impair our ability to remember, think, or make decisions to such a degree that everyday life is impacted.

I assume that if you are reading this book, you already know this. You are well aware of the kind of dementia that your loved one has as well as the symptoms and prognosis.

Have you thought about the assumptions you make that affect how you approach dementia itself?

Did you know that until the 1800s we didn't think about dementia as an illness? Instead, it was considered a natural aspect of aging. In his essay *Framing Confusion: Dementia, Society, and History*, professor Jesse Ballenger explains how we have gone from viewing dementia as a natural state of aging, to a social problem, to a disease that implies catastrophic loss.[4]

Ballenger says that, by the 1930s, government-funded hospitals in the U.S. where people could take advantage of free care were so overrun with supposedly "insane" older adults that, from that point through the mid 1950s, psychologists and social gerontologists began to frame dementia as a social problem. They reasoned that people would be able to compensate for loss of brain function if they had a better living environment. Policies and programs were created to keep the increasing numbers of seniors active and engaged so that their mental abilities could be maintained. With the development of the electron microscope in 1960 and brain imaging techniques in the 1990s, we could zoom in on the plaques and tangles in the brain and began to categorize types of dementia, stages of the disease, and risk factors. Increasingly, as dementia was understood medically, it was positioned as an illness. These developments helped us understand dementia better but, at the same time, funding for research hinged on presenting dementia in the worst possible light. "Advocates represented the losses associated with dementia as so total and irrevocable as to call into question whether people suffering from it could still properly be regarded as people at all, thus greatly deepening the stigmatization of those diagnosed with it and intensifying the anxiety people felt about aging itself," writes Ballenger.[5]

Whether we are aware of it or not, these historical perspectives play in the background of our care. How we think about dementia matters because it dictates how we offer support. It always has. Calling it a mental illness, we warehoused elderly people in hospitals. Viewing it as a social condition, we instituted community programs and policies. Considering it a medical disease, we searched for a cure. We continue to be steeped in a medical model of dementia, and in all the stigma that is informed by the ways of viewing the condition and, by extension, the persons we are caring for.

If we think about dementia in terms of a medical model, we may focus our care exclusively on staving off disease progression and spend our days dragging our loved one from one medical appointment to the next, chasing false cures. If we see caregiving as mostly an individual responsibility, we may not ask for support from family or friends or expect our community to adapt to our needs. If we see illness as entirely negative, we may miss seeing opportunities for deeper connection and expression.

The word dementia itself is loaded. It derives from the Latin. "De" means "lack of" and "ment" has to do with the mind, so *dementia* means "lack of mind." From the get-go, then, people with dementia are defined by what they don't have. As missing something. That idea is cemented into our language (I'll talk about that in the next chapter) and in our assumptions.

What assumptions do you make about dementia, about caregiving, and about illness generally? Do you think of dementia as an all-encompassing disease to be fought, or as another dimension of life? Do you think of it more as a series of losses, or as a potential gateway into a deeper relationship? Is it an inconvenience, a catastrophe, a burden, a blessing?

There is no wrong answer. You might say yes to all of it. In fact, you might feel the burden and blessing keenly in the course of a single day or even a single hour. That's why discernment is so important.

Caring well rests on our ability to discern the ways of framing dementia that are helpful, to analyze our assumptions and sift through mixed messages. The root of the word discern means to separate or sift. As caregivers, we are well acquainted with facing choices. In fact, caring is a series of daily choices. We make small and big choices every day about whether and how much support to give, about how to balance safety concerns with the desire to help our loved one be as independent as possible. In the best of times, making decisions can be hard. Under stress, they can become monumentally difficult. We must bring the best of our intuition, reason, and imagination into our discernment.

Discernment is an inherently spiritual exercise. "What am I going to do?" is a different question than "What action is most in line with the spirit of God's love?" We can think a lot about our decisions and anticipate all the outcomes possible as a result, but spiritual discernment means ensuring God is at the heart of our process.

Each chapter in this book is accompanied by a spiritual exercise aimed to help sharpen our capacity to discern. Why? Because as caregivers, practicing the art of discerning well – sifting between definitions, assumptions, and the stirring of our hearts – can buoy us on the caregiving journey.

To discern, we have to listen. There's a great story about that in the Bible: 1 Kings 19:1–14.

Confronting a king is a bad idea. But what choice did he have? God was leading him – Elijah – to tell King Ahab that he was taking his people in the wrong direction. Now Elijah was running for his life. And he was tired. So very tired. He didn't want to run anymore. He sat under a tree and waited for the king's army to find him. They could do what they wanted to him. He was too tired to care anymore.

Elijah fell into a restless sleep. That's when an angel came, woke him up, and whispered "eat and drink." Astonishingly, Elijah rolled over to find freshly baked bread and hot water. Exhausted, he ate, drank, and fell back asleep. The angel touched him again and said, "Wake up. If you don't get up and eat, the journey will be too much for you." Energized and knowing that the angel was so very near, Elijah made the 40-day journey to Mount Horeb. There, he found a cave and once again drifted off to sleep.

God woke him. "Go out and stand on the mountain."

Outside, the wind ripped around him such that it tore apart rocks. But God wasn't in the wind.

An earthquake erupted beneath Elijah's feet. But God wasn't in the earthquake.

A fire blasted across the mouth of the cave. But God wasn't in the fire.

Then, there was silence.

In a still, small voice, God gave Elijah a new direction for his life.

For over 2,000 years, people of faith have been inspired by Elijah, maybe because his story is so familiar. We all have kings – powerful entities – that dictate our lives; controlling, strong, merciless, exhausting forces we have to confront. For some of us, dementia is one of them.

Elijah's story provides perspective. Dementia doesn't rule our lives – God does. Angels and blessing are always present. There is always bread and water, elements of life that nourish and sustain us. When we are at the end of our rope and feel like we could curl up in a cave somewhere, God reaches into our hearts to forge a tender, sustaining connection, pulling us out of the mire toward a new course of action. When we are fresh out of hope, God introduces us to possibilities we couldn't have imagined for ourselves. We may even find that what we thought was the end wasn't the end after all.

But we have to listen. Pay attention. Tend to our own heart. Because God doesn't always come to us in flashy fires and earthquakes. God comes in silence. In whispers. In a still, small voice.

Caring for someone with dementia often means confronting circumstances we haven't come across before. We need to listen for the still, small voice, especially when "right and wrong" isn't so cut and dried.

Jessie's cheeks glistened, wet with tears. Her husband David bought a brand-new SUV last year. A retired transport driver, he loved nothing more than criss-crossing the country on the open road. Learning that he could no longer drive would be devastating. Telling him so could damage their relationship. Yet Jessie feared for David's safety and the safety of others. "One time, he got so mixed up that he stopped in the middle of a busy highway," she says. "Another time, he intended to go to the post office ten minutes away, left home without his wallet, and wound up lost two hours down the road." Jessie didn't want to go behind her husband's back and tell his doctor or hide his keys. But continuing to do nothing no longer felt right, either. What if he hurt himself? What if he ran over someone? She had weighed all the scenarios and considered various ways to start the conversation. "Have you prayed about it?" I asked.

Pause. "Not really," she said honestly.

We prayed together, holding the whole heap of the dilemma to God. No easy answer came. But Jessie was visibly relieved. She had a power in her corner. One with infinite wisdom and insight. Even though she doubted it would make a difference, Jessie committed to hold up the dilemma to God daily, in prayer, to discern how to broach this difficult subject with her husband.

David saw her praying one day. He asked her what she was doing.

"Really?" David asked, surprised Jessie was talking to God. It was the first time in their married life David had seen Jessie pray. She felt her heart tug. Listening to the still, small voice, she knew that this was the time to be honest with David about her concern around his driving.

"I'm a little bossy," she laughed later in my office. "But I realized in that moment that I shouldn't try to push David into a decision. Instead, I told him how I felt, asked him how he felt, and then asked God to help us discern together what to do next. We never prayed together before. It was weird but nice."

It turns out that seeing Jessie work hard to discern how best to support him inspired David to discern as well. A few weeks later, he gave her the keys.

Not every sticky issue that we discern with God will have a happy ending. Struggle is part of life. Certainty isn't a given. Through our spiritual practices, we draw near to God and trust in God's guidance. The closer we come to God in all our decisions and actions, by listening and by being open and attentive to the nudge of the Spirit, the more centred we will feel no matter the outcome.

"Discernment is a gift of God and simultaneously a habit of faith; although all is grace, there is also, in the mysterious economy of God's plan, a crucial role for human action," writes Elizabeth Liebert in her essay *Discernment for Our Times*. "We choose to notice where God is at work, choose to believe in a larger plan than we can grasp in the moment, choose to hope in the goodness of the future promised by God, choose to align ourselves with God's preferred future as it becomes clear to us."[6] Even when it seems God is absent, the Spirit is nudging us along the path of love.

The late theologian George Hermanson called God the "lure to love," believing that God isn't a guy in the sky but a pervasive, dynamic movement of love in our lives. A love we can be in deep relationship with. A love that draws us toward hope, peace, and joy. Discernment means being attentive to the divine lure and aligning ourselves with it.

Discernment means intentionally opening our hearts to the influence of the Spirit, asking God to help us sort through the information and options before us.

Caregivers are rarely still. Spiritual practice, however, trains our hearts to be still enough through our days to be open to the Spirit.

Through our spiritual practice, we grow more aware of who we are as caregivers and of how we participate in love's great unfolding.

SCRIPTURE: MATTHEW 13:3–9

And he told them many things in parables, saying: "Listen! A sower went out to sow. And as he sowed, some seeds fell on the path and the birds came and ate them up. Other seeds fell on rocky ground, where they did not have much soil, and they sprang up quickly, since they had no depth of soil. But when the sun rose, they were scorched; and since they had no root, they withered away. Other seeds fell among thorns, and the thorns grew up and choked them. Other seeds fell on good soil and brought forth grain, some a hundredfold, some sixty, some thirty. Let anyone with ears listen!"

QUESTIONS FOR REFLECTION AND DISCUSSION

1. Listening is central to discernment in Elijah's story and in this parable, which begins with a command to listen. When do you intentionally listen to discern where God is leading you as you care?
2. How is this parable an exercise in discernment?
3. When do the seeds of your care fall on the path, the rocky ground, the thorns, and the good soil?
4. Where do you see the grain, the benefit of your care? When have the benefits surprised you?

SPIRITUAL PRACTICE: SACRED LISTENING

Similar to *lectio divina*, a traditional monastic practice of reading scripture contemplatively, this spiritual practice is an intentional way of listening to God through scripture. Whether you have ten minutes or a half hour, what's most important is that you choose a time and place to practice sacred listening when you are most likely to hear the call of Love.

1. Read the parable of the sower slowly three times, listening for a word or phrase that speaks to you.
2. Reflect on the word or phrase in silence.
3. Read the passage again three times.
4. Contemplate why you are drawn to those words.
5. Read the passage again three times.
6. How do those words speak to your life right now?
7. Spend time in silence.
8. Give thanks for your insights.

PRAYER

O God, I know that there is a time for everything:

a time to help and a time to refrain from helping,

a time to leap to action and a time to wait patiently,

a time to care for others and a time to care for myself,

a time to be busy and a time to rest,

a time to make decisions and a time to discern a direction,

a time to speak and a time to listen,

a time to name wrongs and a time to admit I'm wrong,

a time to seek joy and a time to be found by it.

Please, God, instill in me the wisdom to know what time this is

and help me make the most of it.

Amen.

3
Realizing You Are a Caregiver

"I don't feel like me. I remind myself
that I still am.
I'm kind of becoming a new me."
– Barb

Jane was still reeling. She and her father had taken her mother for surgery. "I told Dad to stay in the waiting room while I went to move the car. When I got back ten minutes later, he was gone. I freaked. The hospital was huge. I thought I'd never find him," she says. Then, out of the corner of her eye, Jane caught sight of her dad at the far end of the hall. His arm was locked around a nurse's. "He told me she was helping him find Mom," Jane said, adding, "He didn't remember she was in surgery."

The incident was followed by a flood of unwelcome epiphanies. My dad can't be left alone. How did I mistake my mother's corrections and prompts for typical marital cajoling? Am I the parent now?

In an astonishing blink, Jane was suddenly and unexpectedly thrust into the role of caregiver. It was just the beginning of many changes that would affect her relationship with her parents, her role in the family, and how she saw herself.

The Greek philosopher Heraclitus is widely credited with saying, "Change is the only thing constant in life." It's true. Especially when applied to caregiving.

Caregiving is an ever-changing journey shaped by transition. It changes not just what we do but how we think of ourselves. Caregiving shapes and is shaped by our identity.

Identity is what makes you, you. Your identity is formed by the roles you play along with the meanings and expectations you associate with them.

I am, for example, a minister, writer, fundraiser, and caregiver. I'm a parent, daughter, sister, and artist. These roles form my overall identity. Within them, I play other roles and all of them come with expectations.

In my role as a parent, I am a provider, cheerleader, adviser, and more times than I'd wish, a referee. I also have expectations about what it means to be a good provider, cheerleader, adviser ...

Ruth is one the Hebrew Bible's most beloved caregivers. Her identity, as well as the identity of her mother-in-law, Naomi, changed as their personal circumstances and relationships shifted. The story begins with a series of tragic losses.

A famine had already forced them to leave home and now, Ruth and Naomi's husbands have both died. Scripture doesn't explain the cause of death, but it does underscore how palpable their grief is. Naomi changes her name to "Mara," which means bitterness. In ancient times, a person's name reflected their identity. When she changed her name,

Naomi told the world that bitterness and grief overcame all of who she was. In those days, a woman's identity was connected to the men in her life; if a woman wasn't someone's daughter, wife, or mother, she wasn't valued. Feeling acutely empty, Naomi told her two daughters-in-law to leave her and go back to their own families and communities. She knew they no longer had a future with her; they would be childless foreigners if they stayed, their survival uncertain. In that moment, however, Ruth was prepared to leave her family identity behind to assume a new one in Naomi's community as her companion and caregiver. In the longest monologue in the whole book of Ruth, she formalizes the acceptance of her new identity in a pledge.

Do not press me to leave you or to turn back from following you! Where you go, I will go; where you lodge, I will lodge; your people shall be my people, and your God my God. Where you die, I will die – there will I be buried. May the Lord do thus and so to me, and more as well, if even death parts me from you! (Ruth 1:16–17)

At some point, you said to yourself, "I'm a caregiver." Maybe it happened in a moment of crisis. Likely, it was a slower, less conscious progression – one responsibility leading to another until you woke up one day and realized you were a caregiver.

When did you begin to think of yourself as a "caregiver"? Can you pinpoint the moment? Or did it emerge more gradually? You have other identities, too. What are they?

Throughout our lives, some identities come to the fore and others fade. Ruth was a wife and a daughter-in-law among other things. When her husband died, she made a decision to be Naomi's companion and caregiver. Have your identities changed over time? Have some ended or become more important while others have fallen away? Has caregiving had an impact? What do you expect of yourself as a caregiver?

Our identities give us a sense of purpose, self-worth, and self-esteem. They are accompanied by a set of roles and expectations of those roles.

I'm a minister. "Caregiver" is one of the roles expected of a minister. In that role, I believe I ought to behave respectfully, generously, and be present when my community needs me. I am also a mother. Mothering forms a key part of my overall identity. As a mother, I believe I should be emotionally and physically available to care for and nurture my children.

Honestly, I feel most "off" in my life when I don't live up to the expectations I place on myself in any given role, or when one role conflicts with another. An emergency at work doesn't stress me out too much on its own, but when it means that I am unable to be present for my children in their daily crises, I can become resentful. Why? Because the expectations that I have of myself in both roles don't jibe. I am most stressed when I'm not who I aspire to be in the life-roles I most value.

We all carry around a set of expectations about how we are to be in specific roles. These expectations come from our families, our community, our cultural context, our religious associations.

What are the roles you play as a caregiver? Are you now a financial planner, a nurse, a pharmacist? A driver or a cook? Name as many roles as you can. Next to the roles, write down your self-expectations. For example, as "the cook," do you expect that you will cook every meal or that each one will be homemade? Does being "the driver" mean that you expect yourself to drive the person you are caring for to every appointment?

How do you feel both about your roles and the expectations you have as you play them? Where did your expectations come from – culture, society, family? How have they shaped you? Would adjustments to either the role or your expectations be helpful? Are there any expectations you need to let go of or adopt?

"A change in [caregiving] tasks means a change in relationship. There's emotional work as tasks change a relationship," explains Dr. Rhonda Montgomery in an online lecture called *Caregiver Identity Discrepancy and Implications for Practice*.[7] Montgomery spent over 30 years zeroing in on caregiver distress, pinpointing when caregivers feel most stressed to help them avoid burnout. "What we have found through our research is that what we commonly believe – the general assumption that the source of caregiver distress is the amount and type of care that the caregiver is providing – simply isn't true when we look at the data," she says. In reality, caregivers feel most distressed when the tasks they perform don't square with their identity.

Bill tells me that he and his wife Gayle always enjoyed their Jacuzzi bathtub. He cherishes the old times they filled the tub to overflowing and submerged intimately under cover of their favourite bubble bath. It's where the pair discussed their day as friends and connected as lovers. Gayle no longer enjoys the tub. It's all Bill can do to coax her into it. The bathroom has stopped being a place of friendship and romance. "It's a minefield," Bill whispers. "I hate being there. I don't feel like a husband anymore. I'm more like a supervisor."

Caregiving tasks had an impact on the way Bill and Gayle relate to each other. Bill grieved no longer being able to connect with his wife in the way they always had. The bathtub is where the identities clashed most. There, Bill saw himself less as a spouse and more as a supervisor. Holding the two identities in that moment became untenable. According to Montgomery, it's moments like these that "you can change what you are doing, change your relationship, or change the sense of who you are."

Bill realized he had choices. He could decide to bathe Gayle and thus assume more of a caregiver identity, shifting his identity as a spouse. Or he could minimize the activities like bathing that made him feel less like a spouse and add more activities that contribute to his sense of what it meant to be a husband.

"In what other activities do you feel connected?" I asked. "We have always enjoyed walking hand-in-hand by the water," he answered. "We could do that more."

Bill continued to grieve the loss of bathing with his wife, but strolls by the lake did give them both a way to exchange love and affection. Staying emotionally connected felt good. At the same time, Bill hired a homecare worker to attend to the bathing task where the caregiver role particularly grated his spousal one. This helped him focus on ways that drew them closer as spouses.

Changes in day-to-day caregiving tasks and routines can redefine our relationships. Map a timeline of shifts in caregiving responsibilities that had an impact on your self-identity. Next to each significant event, write three words that describe your feelings. When you look at the whole timeline, do you see common patterns or feelings? Share your timeline with a trusted friend, professional confidant, or support group to help provide perspective and reassurance.

"I've become a stranger to myself," Beth told me. She catalogued the changes: there are fewer coffee outings with girlfriends; there is no free time to paint or organize Amnesty International campaigns, and most of the time she is too exhausted at the end of the day to even call her son. Despite being a master gardener, the outside beds are a mess of weeds and the beloved houseplants have all died, save one. "I don't know when it happened. I don't know who I am anymore. I'm certainly not a gardener."

Sometimes, caregiving can become our all-consuming identity. That's okay if we are intentionally choosing to bring that identity to the fore, let other ones go, or at least are at peace with the space caregiving occupies. Sometimes, though, like Beth, we wake up one day to realize that we have totally set aside our own ambitions, dreams, and interests so much so that we struggle to know who we are outside of the caregiving role. We become strangers to ourselves.

Beth's days were filled with countless chores: medical appointments, meals, laundry. Exhausted, she recognized that she was about to hit a wall. "If I lose it, Jim will lose out," she told me. We considered all the tasks she was doing and decided to drop a couple to make space to nurture her own identity as a gardener. She enlisted the help of a good friend to look after Jim three hours a week so that she could be outside in the flower beds. Over time, she enlisted more support and stretched the hours to five.

Aside from being a caregiver, what other identities and roles are important to you right now? Regular journalling can offer a helpful window into how your caregiving experiences are having an impact on who you are becoming. If you feel like you are losing pieces of your identity that you value in the midst of caregiving, try keeping track of when you feel most like yourself in any given day. Being aware of those moments can help you identify the thoughts and activities that can help lead you back to yourself. Self-awareness is key to weaving meaning into our lives as caregivers so that we can find ourselves in our caring role rather than losing ourselves to it.

Caring for Naomi wasn't filled with the toil and trouble Ruth anticipated even though she was quite prepared to make the sacrifices. Caring wasn't a one-way street, either. Naomi's desire to care for Ruth led her to play the role of matchmaker, suggesting that Ruth meet Boaz, a wealthy landowner whom she eventually married. Together, they had a son named Obed.

Naomi, no longer "Mara," became a grandmother. The women in her community blessed her: "And may he [Naomi's grandson] be to you a restorer of life and a nourisher of your old age; for your daughter-in-law, who loves you, who is better to you than seven sons, has borne him" (Ruth 4:15).

Naomi grew so close to the boy and he to her that some spoke of Naomi as his second mother. Obed would grow up to have children of his own who also had children. One of them was King David. Back when her husband died and Naomi became destitute and so thoroughly depressed that she changed her name to Mara, she wouldn't have imagined that one day she would become the great-grandmother of a king.

Caring is an extension of God's grace. It can't help but change us in ways we don't anticipate. While some of our roles rise and fall and our sense of who we are shifts, our identity as one of God's "beloved" is constant.

Whatever else you are, you are a child of God. That means the love of God's very self is born within you. Rest in that love. Care from that place of love. Regard yourself as God would. Know that God is working through you and all of who you are to bless and love. Identities shift and roles come and go, but faith, hope, and love abide, and the greatest of these is love.

SCRIPTURE: RUTH 1:16

But Ruth said, "Do not press me to leave you or to turn back from following you! Where you go, I will go; where you lodge, I will lodge; your people shall be my people, and your God my God."

QUESTIONS FOR REFLECTION AND DISCUSSION

1. Who do you identify with most: Ruth, Naomi, Boaz, Obed? Why?
2. What identities and roles have changed in your life? Which have remained constant?
3. When have you felt you needed to shift your expectations related to your roles, or needed to let go of a role? What happened when you did?
4. Who or what has had the biggest influence in shaping the expectations you have of yourself as a caregiver?

SPIRITUAL PRACTICE: DRAWING REFLECTION

Don't worry! You don't need any artistic skill for this spiritual practice. You simply have to be able to make two lines. Any writing tool and piece of scrap paper will do.

1. Very slowly, begin to draw a street anywhere on the bottom of your page. The street begins at the start of your life.

2. With each major move or transition in your life, alter the road accordingly. Were you at a crossroads during those transitions, were you just gently curving, or did you have to slam on the brakes, bend, or do a 180? Beside each transition, write the ways your identity, roles, and expectations shifted. Continue to draw your road until it brings you to today.

3. Now add feelings to those transitions. How did you feel then? How do you feel now?

4. Where did you sense God in those times?

5. As you look at the road, what are the common themes?

6. Where did you find strength? What did you learn about change?

7. What spiritual learning could you apply to changes you are experiencing now?

8. Ask God to bless your journey.

PRAYER

I am many things, but first and foremost I am your child, Holy One –
Created in your image, my caring is instinctive,
an embedded, divine impulse to love.
Through all of life's transitions, you are there
beckoning me on the journey,
shaping me all the while.
Through change and uncertainty,
I know your heart beats strong within me,
blessing me to care in concert with you.
Thank you.
Amen.

4

Challenging Assumptions and Stigma

"There are a lot of people who hide at home
when they're diagnosed, who don't share their story.
If I have dementia, I'm going to be open about it –
when I'm out talking to someone and mix up my words,
I'll just explain that I have dementia."
– Ken, *a national ambassador for
the Canadian Alzheimer's Society*[8]

She wasn't about to accept "no." Her daughter was sick and she desperately needed help. Like any of us would, the Syrophoenician mother in Mark's gospel (Mark 7:24–30) was prepared to do whatever it took to make sure her daughter got the care she needed. But it wasn't natural for Jews and Syrophoenicians to mix, given the longstanding discord between Jews and Gentiles. Jesus responded to her request for help by telling her that his care was reserved for Israelites. The mother pressed him. She emphatically told Jesus that his view of care was too narrow and that he needed to expand his perspective. Her argument was convincing. Jesus healed her daughter.

Stigma, like the kind the Syrophoenician woman in Mark's gospel faced, can be a serious issue for people with dementia. For some, like Norman, the impact of stigma is worse than the condition itself.

Norman was growing more and more reserved during the coffee time after church. Three years earlier, he would mingle amongst the huddles of congregants, gregariously chatting about his latest trip to the cottage or the new restaurant in town. Gradually, he had become introverted and withdrawn. "I'm not sure if what I'll say is right," he told me when I mentioned he didn't seem to be joining in quite as much. "If I say anything, they'll think of me differently," he said. "If I don't say much, I won't say anything wrong."

Norman didn't fear saying the wrong thing, he feared how people would see him if he did. For many, the deepest stress of dementia isn't the disease, it's that others will think less of them and they will be ashamed of who they are.

Stigma is a serious issue with serious impacts. It can result in a decision not to seek an early diagnosis that could help manage symptoms. It can also leave people suddenly isolated and lonely.

Caregivers can help.

We all form our sense of self-worth, at least in part, from how others regard us. The stigma-free care we provide can convey worth, comfort, and belonging for the person we care for, and can influence wider networks to be more care-full.

As caregivers, we are like mirrors. Through the quality of our care, those we care for perceive their sense of worth. That's good news because it means that when we hold up a stigma-free mirror through our care, we can convey comfort and belonging.

But we don't care in a vacuum any more than Jesus did. Outside prejudice can seep into our perceptions. As a caregiver, you may have not only have experienced the stigma of dementia but absorbed it, too. Maybe even unconsciously.

Every second, we process approximately 200,000 times more information unconsciously than we do consciously.[9] That's why it's so important to examine our beliefs and assumptions intentionally. Our assumptions lead to decisions that ultimately lead to helpful or unhelpful thoughts and actions.

Contentment in our caregiving roles, not to mention the well-being of the person we are caring for, hinge on big ideas about what it means to be a person. Society teaches us that having value as a human being requires us to have brains that fire "normally." That's a devastating perspective for people with dementia because it ultimately means they are becoming less of a person as their brain changes.

Caring well for people with dementia requires us to challenge the perspective that reason trumps other important human experiences in life, such as belonging, loving, and being loved.

The idea that our ability to reason is our most valuable asset is hard to dislodge because the perspective runs more than half a century deep.

The philosophical proposition issued by French philosopher René Descartes (1596–1650) "I think, therefore I am" has shaped our understanding of what it means to be a person since the mid-17th century. Descartes didn't mean that thought and *being* are fundamentally the same thing, but that's how he was understood. On the heels of

Descartes, philosopher John Locke (1632–1704) wrote that being a person is "to be a thinking, intelligent being that has reason and reflection."[10]

These philosophies so firmly planted in Western thought equate what it means to be a person with typical brain function. They marry having value with the ability to reason. The flip side of these ideas about personhood means that people who do not have the capacity to reason or remember are deemed less than human.

"Not all there" is the derogatory expression popularly used to describe neurological difference. "Not all there" equates "being there" or rather "here, fully alive in the now" with the ability to reason.

I've heard many caregivers refer to their loved one as a "shell" of their former selves, "not fully with it" or "not there at all." This kind of language means we have internalized stigma and it jeopardizes our ability to care well. Why? Because absence and shells don't merit care – fully alive beings do.

If we understand dementia as a disintegration of who we are until we are an empty vessel, or a non-person, then there is less motivation to understand, empathize, and offer care. If we as caregivers buy into this philosophy, we may find ourselves trying to hide the impact of the disease from those around us. Sometimes, we do this at the expense of our own well-being and to the detriment of our loved one, who may benefit from an earlier diagnosis. Also, in moments of high stress, stigma may filter through our words.

What do you think makes you, you? Surely, you are more than your memory or even your brain synapses. That's not to say memory isn't important, but memory isn't *all* of what makes us who we are. What makes us who we are flows through the world, as well as through and between every person. In fact, I think we become who we are through relationships.

For as long as I can remember, I've been told that I'm creative and determined, so much so that I've not only come to believe it, but that self-image has guided my approach to life. Many times when I've been on the verge of quitting something, I've reminded myself that quitting isn't in my nature. When I've found myself in a bind, I've called on my creativity to be resourceful. Outside voices that I have internalized have shaped me as much as anything else.

The idea that outside voices and influences play an important role in shaping who we are as individuals means that we, as caregivers, have an incredible opportunity. It means that you and I are uniquely positioned to help someone with dementia maintain their sense of self, experience the world, and create meaning. Caregivers have the profound capacity to "re-member" a person. In other words, we have the ability to help the people we care for reconnect with who they are, and, in the process, we may even reconnect with who we are.

Marie's voice broke. Her hand shook visibly as I passed her a cup of coffee. Her husband had just received a diagnosis of Alzheimer's. It's not that Marie hadn't already anticipated what the doctor was going to say or that she herself hadn't pressed for a diagnosis. But now it just seemed so final. "I'm just not ready for everything to slip away. For Jim to be an empty shell ... gone. For me to ... " her voice trailed off.

I encouraged her to finish her sentence.

"For me to slip away, too," she said.

"Why do you think that's going to happen?" I asked.

"It happened to my mother," she replied.

Marie's father had Alzheimer's and her mother cared for him. As Marie saw it, the disease took over her mother's life until she had none left.

"From now on, there will be three people in our life – Jim, me, and Alzheimer's and soon there will be one," she said.

Marie was making several assumptions: that her mother's experience would be her own, that Alzheimer's was in control, and that ultimately it would result in both her and Jim becoming an empty shell of themselves.

Joining an online support group helped Marie challenge her assumptions. She met people there who had good days and bad days and yet found caregiving to be a meaningful call. She found ways to be in control, to feel that she and Jim were determining their future. She developed a support system to lean on and found a quality of friendship that she had never before experienced. She began to identify and nurture facets of life that weren't affected by Alzheimer's. Beneath it all, she broadened her understanding of what it means to be human.

"I wouldn't trade it," she told me a couple of years later. "I never thought I'd say there was anything positive in this, but there is. I see the world in a whole new way now. I wouldn't go so far as to say dementia is a gift, but I have found gifts through the experience."

Some commentators don't like the story about the Syrophoenician woman in Mark because they think it portrays Jesus as weak at best, and prejudicial at worst, but I think it's one of the Bible's most beautiful stories. I don't mind that Jesus wasn't always perfect. His legacy to us isn't perfection, it's that in moments of imperfection, he consistently expanded his heart. Wrestling with our identity, roles, assumptions, and perspectives is deeply faithful. It's the very well from which emotional and spiritual growth springs.

Each time I visited Alita, I found her cradling a plastic doll, cooing and rubbing its blonde hair. One day, I made the mistake of reaching out to touch it. Alita looked at me squarely in the eyes – the first time she had done so over the months that I had visited – and hissed angrily. I didn't have permission to touch her baby. Alita was being a good mother, protecting her child from me, a stranger.

Although well into her 80s, motherhood was the world Alita was living in. I intruded rudely, and despite not being able to use words, Alita let me know precisely what she thought.

The next time I visited her, I brought my own son with me. He was just five months old at the time. I showed Alita my baby. I talked about being a first-time mother and the trials and tribulations of caring for a little one. I told her I thought she was a good mother herself and that I hoped to be one too. I sang the lullaby I sing to my son. It was the most relaxed I had ever seen her. She happily reached out and stroked my son's arm. We connected – as mothers. What an honour it was to sit in the presence of someone who had been such a good mother and who took her maternal role seriously. Alita was a mother-bear until the end of her life; I aspire to be such a devoted parent.

Looking back, I realize I hadn't asked permission to touch Alita's baby and hadn't provided any physical cues that I was going to do so. I also hadn't tried to enter Alita's reality, thinking of the doll as an inanimate object rather than as Alita's lifeblood.

While my caregiving methods might not have been well-honed, my intentions were good. I have always strived to let spiritual values guide my care although admittedly, sometimes I've fallen short.

"Dignity" stems from the French word *dignite*. From this word comes "dignitary." That's how I like to think about the care I give. My way of caring should strive to be intentional and honouring, each action respectfully valuing the person I'm caring for.

For me, that means trying to meet people where they are. When I'm caring for people with dementia in particular, it means striving to communicate in ways they feel are meaningful, supporting them to be as independent as they want to be, recognizing each person's uniqueness, and viewing myself as a learner.

What values and principles guide your caregiving? Write down a list of values that spring to mind. Reflect on each word. How do you live these out? Are there any instances where these values come into conflict with each other?

Admittedly, one of the values I've struggled with most is helping. I am guessing that you, like me, were raised to be helpful. Being helpful is a lovely trait. Many caregivers are natural "do-ers." That said, I have learned that caring sometimes means less *doing* and more *being*. For instance, one time, I leapt to open a soft drink for a congregant I was visiting, "helpfully" pouring it into the cup and hastily inserting a straw at the first awkward pause. It felt good to do something to help.

Today I realize I'm most helpful when I support self-sufficiency. Sometimes that means holding back. I'll wait to see if the person is inclined to perform a task like opening a can themselves. If there is no movement, I'll raise the can and say, "Here's some pop if you would like it" and wait for verbal or bodily acknowledgement before I open it.

All of us want to be in control of our lives and to make choices for ourselves. Our sense of quality of life is connected to the power we have to guide it. Caregivers should seek to acknowledge, respect, and restore power rather than assume it. Sometimes, people with dementia can't initiate a task, but once they get started a kind of muscle-memory takes over. Prompts can help.

Try breaking the task at hand into steps and prompting the steps: for example, opening the can, pouring the drink into the cup, placing a straw in the cup. Initiating the task by helping someone to pick up the straw and then stepping back while they complete the job can support their desire to be as independent as possible.

Whether it is pouring a drink, completing a task related to personal hygiene, or going on an outing, fostering dignity in our care means focusing on the abilities of the person we are with rather than on what the person *can't* do. That's important because how we think and feel about ourselves is so often tied to the way we think others perceive us. If, as caregivers, we too quickly leap to accomplish a task for the person we are caring for, we run the risk of making them feel inadequate, reinforcing one of the deepest fears those living with dementia have – that others will think less of them. If that fear becomes established, ultimately, they will think less of themselves.

Over time, I've become more attuned to my "why's" and more comfortable asking myself humbling questions: Why is it easier for me to "help" than to take a wait-and-see approach? Am I leaping to help because my help is needed, or is it because I can't abide the struggle, or because I'm impatient, or because I like to be needed? What values and assumptions penetrate my care?

"Know thyself," sounds cliché, but leaning into why we do what we do – our impulses and motives – can sharpen our compassion.

What has caregiving taught you?

No doubt, you have been changed by it. Caregiving is nothing if not a journey of learning and growth. It is a path marked by as many questions as answers, if not more. Lean into the questions. The best ones can expand the direction of our care if not the trajectory of our lives.

If the Syrophoenician woman hadn't been so insistent, if she hadn't probed and questioned Jesus' views, exposed the way he bought into stigma, and if Jesus hadn't been open enough to allow her rebuke to expand his heart, nothing else would have followed. He wouldn't have criss-crossed the ancient world preaching love to anyone who would listen. He wouldn't have made himself available to care for the least and the lost. Thank God she spoke up. Thank God Jesus listened.

SCRIPTURE: MARK 7:25–30

[B]ut a woman whose little daughter had an unclean spirit immediately heard about him, and she came and bowed down at his feet. Now the woman was a Gentile, of Syrophoenician origin. She begged him to cast the demon out of her daughter. He said to her, "Let the children be fed first, for it is not fair to take the children's food and throw it to the dogs." But she answered him, "Sir, even the dogs under the table eat the children's crumbs." Then he said to her, "For saying that, you may go – the demon has left your daughter." So she went home, found the child lying on the bed, and the demon gone.

QUESTIONS FOR REFLECTION AND DISCUSSION

1. When have you encountered stigma around dementia? How has it affected you and the person you are caring for?
2. What questions/situations have challenged you on your journey with dementia? How have you grown as a person?
3. What values inform how you care?
4. Where can you see your relationship with God expanding as a result of your caregiving?

SPIRITUAL PRACTICE: SENSING GOD'S ETERNAL LIGHT

1. Light a candle. It can be a battery-operated one or a regular candle. If you don't have one, draw near to a window with good light, or to a lamp whose light is a comfort.
2. Notice the tense areas in your body and begin to relax them.
3. Imagine the light from your candle or lamp entering your body. It is God's light. As it makes its way from your head to your toes, imagine it flushing out stress, washing away fatigue, strengthening your muscles.
4. Dwell in the light.
5. Now imagine the light is pouring out from you and washing over the one you are caring for so that they, too, are bathed in God's light.

6.   Imagine extending the light to others: family, friends, neigh-
     bours, care workers. They, too, radiate with God's light.

7.   Imagine the light going from you and your loved ones into the
     world, streaming across the grass, the trees, the streets, the
     buildings ...

8.   Pray: May the light of grace enlighten me and flow through me,
     Holy One. May each person I meet experience your grace in me,
     and may I experience you wherever I go and whatever I do.
     Amen.

ONE-MINUTE PRAYER

I only have a minute, God,

and I want to spend it breathing deeply of your Spirit.

I breathe in your peace and breathe out my anxiety.

I breathe in your grace and breathe out my anger.

I breathe in your love and breathe out my desire for revenge.

I breathe in your hope and breathe out my despair.

I breathe in your energy and breathe out my fatigue.

I breathe in your openness and breathe out my judgments.

I breathe in your abundance and breathe out my emptiness.

I breathe in your joy and breathe out my cynicism.

I breathe deeply of your light, O God.

I am always amazed at what you can accomplish in me in just a minute.

Amen.

5
Loving with and without Words

"Hi Rita, it's Reverend Trish from the church," I said, sitting down.

Rita began stroking the back of my hand.

A moment later, she wrapped my hands in hers and

nuzzled them against her neck.

"It's good to see you, too, Rita," I responded.

The prodigal son rehearsed. He had boldly asked for his inheritance early, travelled, blew through the family money, and when he was literally starving, decided it would be best to return home. Tail firmly between his legs, he rehearsed what he would say to get back into his father's good graces: "Father, I have sinned against heaven and against you. I am no longer worthy to be called your son; make me like one of your hired servants" (Luke 15:11–20, paraphrase).

Have you ever rehearsed what you were going to say? How about replaying what you did say because you didn't have time to rehearse, or it just came out wrong? We rehearse because we know our words matter. Words can mend, divide, conquer, evade. They can become hurtful weapons or helpful tools of love.

We use language to communicate and forge relationships, to give voice to our thoughts and experiences. In the process, language determines our reality. When we hear harsh words, for example, we may feel unloved, which might then make us behave as though we are not loved.

Our assumptions about dementia and caregiving are evident in our language. Stigma can be betrayed in our words. Which is why we need to pay attention to them.

Too often, we infantilize people with dementia without even being conscious of it. For example, the language we use to describe our caregiving frequently derives from experiences in our families, particularly raising children. We use language like "babysitting" to describe our presence with the person, and "diapers" and "bibs" to describe items we use to support our care.

These are the kinds of terms we need to resist if we aspire to nurture the dignity of the people we care for. While we may be tempted to think it doesn't matter which words we use because the person will not be able to recall them, feelings last. We may forget the precise nature of the sticks and stones, but none of us forget how they make us feel.

The same goes for how we talk to persons with dementia. If we don't have an intimate relationship with the person we are caring for, referring to him or her as "sweetheart," "dear," or "honey," is patronizing. Asking "How are *we* doing today?" rather than "How are *you* doing today?" implies that the person we are caring for doesn't have a sense of identity as an individual.

Studies tell us that adults who are spoken to as children can begin to doubt their own ability, are more likely to resist care, and can become less communicative.[11] When we talk to people with dementia, we always need to speak with respect.

Of course, we may need to alter our communication style as new symptoms arise. For some people with dementia, providing concrete examples rather than asking an open-ended question can be helpful. We can, for example, reframe the question "What do you want to do today?" by providing options: "Would you like to watch a movie or go to the mall?" Asking questions that can be responded to with "yes" or "no" can be useful when the person we are caring for may understand the question but not have the linguistic ability to respond. The beauty of "yes" and "no" questions in these situations is that feelings can be communicated through a nod or shake of the head.

There may be times when we need to change the volume of our voice, speak more slowly, repeat, rephrase, or draw physically close to communicate more effectively. Still, when we change our approach, it needs to be in the interest of supporting a person's independence and dignity.

When I was in public school, one of my teachers was fond of randomly calling on students to answer math questions. She wrote a formula on the board and then called our name. We had to stand beside our desks and announce our answer in front of the entire class. Numbers were never my strong suit. The whole exercise, likely intended to sharpen our numeric skills, was a lesson in humiliation. I wished the floor would swallow me whole.

That memory sprung to mind as I was getting ready to preside at Norm's celebration of life.

The family was gathering outside the chapel with Norman's wife,

Jean, who had Alzheimer's. One of Jean's children introduced me to her. I said hello and that I was glad to meet her. "We're here for Dad's funeral, Mom," one of her daughters told her in an uncomfortably loud voice. She grasped her mother's arm and spun her around. "Do you remember Dad, Mom?"

Jean was obviously uncomfortable. She didn't want to lie and didn't know the answer. "I ... I ... she stammered."

Her daughter continued. "Norman ... Dad, Mom. Do you know who I'm talking about?"

Jean didn't answer. Her daughter turned to me and said, "Mom's really not with it today," then turned back to Jean and said, "Norm is Dad, Mom."

It might be tempting to test our loved one's cognition by quizzing them, especially in situations where we feel stressed. We so long for our loved ones to have the answer! But quizzes, especially public ones, can heap shame on those we are caring for.

Testing questions such as "What year did we open the cottage?" or memory-related questions such as "Do you remember when?" risk communicating failure more than love. Instead, consider turning the question into an answer, providing the information rather than putting the person on the spot: "I remember the time we went camping and you ate all the chocolate for the s'mores."

Corrections can be as painful as quizzes. If our loved one expresses something that we know to be factually wrong, it's usually best not to correct them. What's the point of highlighting their memory issue unless their faulty idea could cause harm? Most of the time, it's best to focus on being compassionate rather than accurate, positive rather than negative.

Reminisce. Tell stories of fun times. Chat about changes in the family, or what's happening in the neighbourhood. Laugh when it feels right. Describe where you are, the view outside, or the flowers in the foyer. Be truly present and open to moments of joy. Express appreciation for your loved one.

There may come a time when our loved one can't converse in typical ways through language because dementia can damage the language centres of the brain. Damage can result in problems like finding the right words, substituting words, and using the wrong sequence of words.[12]

Losing the ability to communicate through words can be really difficult and traumatic for both the caregiver and the person with dementia. Rest assured that it isn't the end of the world, though. Your care is about love. And love always speaks.

When he was still a distance off, the prodigal son could make out a figure running toward him. Who is that? Could it be? The prodigal's mouth slacked. It's my father!

In his time and culture, grown men didn't run. Yet here was his father, not just running, but running to meet *him*! The prodigal's steps quickened on instinct. Soon, he too was running flat out. A few months ago, he ran away to experience his own life; now he was running home to save it. No words were needed. The dusty, breathless embrace said it all (Luke 15:20, paraphrase).

When you can no longer rely on words to help build and sustain your care, there is an opportunity to develop new skills with which to speak the language of love. Positively, this means we can open ourselves to new modes of self-expression. We are already acquainted with some of these modes, if subconsciously. Nonverbal communication techniques are not only available to us, they are embedded in our bodies and habits.

American anthropologist Ray Birdwhistell pioneered the first study of nonverbal communication in the late 1940s. He observed that while the average person only speaks for a total of ten to 11 minutes a day, we can make and recognize over 200,000 facial expressions.[13] Dementia can't diminish the power of love. Expressing it means tuning in.

Be intentional and attentive to your body language. Are you physically open? Do you appear truly interested in the person you are caring for? Do your actions and tone reveal what you intend to communicate? What about the environment you are trying to communicate in? Is there too much distraction? Is any background noise hindering your ability to relate?

Experiment with different ways of caring non-verbally, taking the nature of your relationship with the person you are caring for into account. If it's appropriate, hold their hand. Offer a foot or hand massage. Pat their back. Place a warm towel over their feet or shoulders. Go for a walk arm in arm. Fix a warm or cool drink. Give a hug. Make sure to look for signs that they are comfortable and stop if it seems they aren't.

Early in my ministry, when I cared for people with late-stage dementia, I was at a loss. Far from embracing an opportunity to develop new communication skills, I felt uneasy, frustrated, and even kind of useless. If the person couldn't acknowledge my presence, would my visit make any difference? What kind of relationship could I develop through a totally one-sided conversation?

Rick was the first person with Alzheimer's I cared for as a minister. He was unable to speak. I struggled to find topics to broach. More often than not, he wheeled away his chair as I awkwardly searched for something to say. Mentors encouraged me to reach out to his family and ask them about his interests so I could make a plan for my visit. From them I learned that Rick liked Westerns, so I brought along a Western novel to read aloud. A staff member told me Rick was a fan of country music, especially Johnny Cash. So, another visit, I brought along "Rock Island Line" and hummed along. I noticed a trend. When Rick was interested, he'd stick around and when he wasn't, he would wheel away. We were communicating! Rick shared what he liked and disliked very effectively. He voted with his feet. No words required.

Rick taught me an important lesson. Just because a person with dementia can't speak to you doesn't mean they don't know what they want. Communication never stops, even in later stages of dementia. Instead, it becomes nonverbal, continuing through sounds, as well as movements like pointing, tapping, breathing heavily, and moving eyes.[14] Being attentive to the body language of the person – which may indicate that they are in discomfort or pain, or point to what continues to matter most to them – can help us build relationships with them. Memory and meaning are not only stored in our mind but in our body, too.

David spent so long bowing by his bed, his forehead bobbing down, that his back hurt. Each time staff found David bent over, they tried to coax him to lay down. One day, I heard him recite words to the Lord's Prayer and I realized he was praying. In fact, every time I noticed he was bent over, he said these words. Later, I learned from family members that David was raised a devout Christian. While he could no longer find all the words to pray, his body assumed the position. David's body communicated who he was (a person of faith) and what he needed (comfort and connection with the divine) long after words eluded him.

The risk in chalking bodily behaviour we don't understand up to confusion on the part of the person with dementia rather than our own lack of understanding is that our well-meaning care may be misdirected, and we may miss opportunities to reinforce our loved one's sense of self or meaningful interactions.

Shortly after I suggested to David's niece Rebecca that he might be praying, she began to pray with him. Praying alongside her uncle was profoundly meaningful and life changing for her. As she recognized how important faith was to David, she re-discovered her own faith. David's witness changed her life.

In order to live well, human beings require food, water, shelter, sleep, and relationships with others. Relationships aren't built on language. Yes, our words matter. But they aren't everything. Our physical presence matters, too. As caregivers, we ourselves are the message, and the message is love. The beautiful irony is that when we embody love, we often find ourselves on the receiving end of it.

His arm still around his prodigal son, the father called the servants. "Quick! Bring the best robe and put it on him. Put a ring on his finger and sandals on his feet."

In his time and culture, people would have expected the father to beat his son for that kind of insolence. Instead, the father called for a celebration, gathering the community for a welcome-home meal.

"Bring the fattened calf and kill it. Let's have a feast and celebrate. For this son of mine was dead and is alive again; he was lost and is found." So they began to celebrate (Luke 15:22–24, paraphrased).

Probably some spoke. Probably some didn't. No matter. There was food, music, and dancing. Universal languages through which we love.

SCRIPTURE: LUKE 15:20–24

So he set off and went to his father. But while he was still far off, his father saw him and was filled with compassion; he ran and put his arms around him and kissed him. Then the son said to him, "Father, I have sinned against heaven and before you; I am no longer worthy to be called your son." But the father said to his slaves, "Quickly, bring out a robe – the best one – and put it on him; put a ring on his finger and sandals on his feet. And get the fatted calf and kill it, and let us eat and celebrate; for this son of mine was dead and is alive again; he was lost and is found!" And they began to celebrate.

QUESTIONS FOR REFLECTION AND DISCUSSION

1. In what ways do you express the "languages of love" in the way you care?
2. How can you be more attentive to your own body language and to the body language of the person for whom you are caring?

3. List the ways you offer care without words. Of these, which do you consider most important?
4. How is the father in the story of the prodigal son a model of care?

SPIRITUAL PRACTICE: CONTEMPLATIVE WALK

In scripture, God's people are always on the move. The Israelites walked to the promised land, Abram and Noah were lauded for walking with God, and the risen Christ appeared to the disciples as they walked along the Emmaus road. In the parable of the prodigal son, both the father and the son are moving. As the son walks home, the father runs toward him. The point biblical writers underscored is that wherever we go, God is with us.

When we walk contemplatively, we literally "go with God." Contemplative walking is not about arriving at a destination or getting exercise, it's about connecting with the spirit's sacred presence.

1. Go for a walk. Alternatively, move your feet while sitting down or tap your hands on your armrest to emulate footsteps.
2. Walk or tap contemplatively, deliberately. Notice the contact your foot is making with the ground, heel to toe, or if you are using your hand, wrist to fingertip. Slow down. Time the rhythm of your breath to the rhythm of your movement.
3. Ask yourself, "Where in my life do I need to sense God's mercy and compassion?" Spend half of the time you have allotted for this spiritual exercise reflecting on that question as you walk or move.

4. As you turn back toward home for the second half of the journey, invite God to move with you. Sense that the spirit of God is alongside you, walking with you toward home. Feel the presence of God's mercy and compassion. Breathe deeply.

5. As your walk concludes, give thanks to God for being your constant companion.

PRAYER

Make me aware of my thoughts, O God,
   because they inform my words.
Make me aware of my words, O God,
   because they inform my actions.
Make me aware of my actions, O God,
   because they inform my relationships.
Make me aware of my relationships, O God,
   because they inform my being.
Make me aware of my being, O God,
   because I have my being in you.
Make me aware of you, O God,
   make me aware of you.
   Amen.

6

Caring Creatively
through the Arts

"I used to have my Grade 9 piano but I got busy
and haven't played for years. That's changed
since my diagnosis. It's wonderful. I play all the time
now. I perform in concerts. I'm learning ukulele.
I think it's creating new pathways for me."
– Daphne

"What do you do?" is the first question many of us ask when we meet someone new. In the book of Genesis, we meet God for the first time. Creating is what God does. God's creative energy breathes life into our very being and into everything that is.

God's creativity continues to flower, even today, as it flows through us. Creativity is an expression of the divine within us. Creativity is as core to us as breathing. Dementia can't take it away.

An accomplished musician, Stella accompanies hymns during church services at the continuing care centre. Worship takes place in a cramped chapel with little space for residents and wheelchairs much less instruments. There's a pitiful sounding keyboard with a broken pedal while a hair's breadth outside the door sits a grand piano.

Occasionally, Stella leaves the chapel mid-service and sits down on the bench at the piano stationed in the hallway. Each time she does, residents remark that she is growing increasingly confused.

Stella is often disoriented and agitated; she never remembers my name and occasionally forgets her own. Yet when she plays the keyboard during the services, she strikes complex chords from memory. While Stella appears to randomly wander off mid-service, she is actually seeking out the better instrument. Her timing may be awkward, but her instinct is right. Who would want to play a broken-down keyboard when a few feet away there's a grand piano?

How can Stella remember complicated church music and opt for the better instrument yet forget she's playing in the chapel?

Daniel Levitin, professor emeritus at McGill University and author of *This Is Your Brain on Music* tells me over the phone that the changes in the brain that serve to store a memory are called a memory trace. "Music has so many different components that when it forms a memory trace in the brain, there are a lot of different ways that the trace becomes activated. So what I mean is, music has pitch, melody, rhythm, harmony, timbre, maybe words and also feelings associated with the song, especially if you've heard it before. All those things make the memory trace robust," says Levitin.

In other words, because music has an impact on so many parts of the brain, even if one area is negatively affected, the others may still be intact.

The possibility that the arts are a gateway to accessing memory is exciting, but recent research suggests the arts have other benefits too.

For over a decade, the National Gallery of Australia has hosted weekly hour-long tours for people with dementia. For six weeks participants discuss and engage with artwork. Researchers have discovered scientific evidence that the tours change the chemical makeup of the brain.[15]

Normally, the stress hormone cortisol is high when we wake up, decreases during the day, and drops to its lowest point at night. In people with dementia, the rhythm is disrupted causing stress, agitation, and lowering cognition. When researchers tested the saliva of 28 participants in the National Gallery's dementia program before, during, and after joining in, they found cortisol levels improved and generally people reported feeling better.

It's early days and more testing is required, but the anecdotal and scientific evidence is mounting: creativity helps not only to evoke memory but boosts confidence, facilitates communication, supports identity, and builds relationships.

The science has huge implications for caregivers. It means that tapping into creativity can enhance our care.

"But I'm not an artist," you might argue. Never mind that. We don't need to be the next Picasso to create. My favourite quote is by Corita Kent, who was a Roman Catholic nun, pop artist, and advocate: "Creativity belongs to the artist in each of us. To create means to relate. The root meaning of the word art is to fit together, and we all do this every day … Each time we fit things together we are creating – whether it is to make a loaf of bread, a child, a day."[16]

In other words, creativity is baked into who we are so much so that we create without realizing it. We make meals, hang photos, write words, organize objects, hum or sway to music, dig in the garden, doo-dle ... and on and on.

If you don't think of yourself as creative, maybe it's because you have been taught to devalue your creativity. This is what happens to most of us. Over the years, little by little, our sense of ourselves as creative beings is stripped away, and we eventually stop pursuing creative en-deavours as though we are not worthy of them. Think back to grade school when you did arts and crafts. Were you given the end product and graded on your ability to replicate what was effectively someone else's creation?

Society teaches us that being successfully artistic means having the potential to create a product that will sell. There are very few "real art-ists" who cut the mustard to make a living doing it.

What would happen if we decided that creative success is less about the end result and more about the journey? What if we deemed the creative process itself to be the true masterpiece? I'm convinced that the joy we get from putting paint to canvas is or can be as satisfying as deeming it good enough to hang on the wall, and that the pleasure we get from singing to ourselves is as life-giving as performing in a con-cert. How good we feel when we are being creative is as important if not more important than the final product.

For over 25 years I've hosted art workshops, focusing not on the product of creativity but on the process of creation. The objective is to tap into our creativity to expand awareness of ourselves and the spirit.

Helen attended one of my first workshops. I'll never forget her. She stood against a wall, which was covered with a giant piece of craft pa-per, while I traced her form with a dark marker. After we were finished, we went to the art room where I had laid out glue and strips of fabric. Gingerly, Helen stuck one layer of fabric after another after another onto her form. So many layers of clothing!

"Are these layers like armour?" I asked.

Not able to retrieve words, Helen nodded. She began adding square pieces of fabric over her heart area.

"I wonder why you are covering your heart, Helen?" I inquired. "Do you feel you need to protect yourself?" I asked.

No, she shook her head.

"Do people not see your heart?" I asked.

Yes, she nodded.

Over several sessions, Helen shared with me many feelings – anger, loss, sadness. As Helen brought her art to life, she invited me to get to know her better. It was holy ground.

I saw Helen and she felt seen. The art was a means of communication, of sharing, of relationship building. It was invaluable not because it was great art but because it was great expression.

Letting go of the creative outcome and judgment of our art can be a monumental mindset shift. Since the industrial revolution, we have been taught that imagination is less important and useful than reason and facts. Still today, math and the sciences are seen as more valuable than "bird" courses such as visual arts and drama. Fact is prioritized over fiction as though hard news is the best way to share deep truths.

Dr. Anne Basting, pioneer of TimeSlips,[17] a creative approach to dementia care, says that when we ask people with memory loss to remember, we're asking them to go to their place of loss to express themselves. "It's inviting the person into shame and failure. What creativity and imagination demand of us is to let go of that. Certainly, memories come out, because you can't completely separate memory and imagination. But if you let go of the expectation of memory, you open up so many more possibilities," she explains in an interview.[18]

Creativity doesn't depend on memory, learning, or language, and it's a beautiful way of sharing feelings, ideas, and who we are with each other. Making art is one of the ways caregivers can bring joy into people's lives.

What we create always speaks of who we are deep inside. Think about it. Nothing we create can be exactly duplicated. Everything we make is utterly original. Therefore, creativity is an expression of the uniqueness of our deepest self. For people with dementia who feel that they are losing themselves and a sense of their own personhood, being able to express their creativity is powerfully restorative.

We don't need fancy supplies to invite expression and foster connection through creativity. Something as simple as looking at images together can build relationship and rapport.

For years, I have kept a small box in the trunk of my car. It is filled with laminated art images, each about four inches square. When I visit those who cannot speak using words, I ask them if they would like to look at the art with me. I ask them to pick an image that touches their heart. When they choose one, I spend time "noticing" it with them.

On one such visit, Jim picked a Picasso. We spent time noticing the hard angles, vibrant colours, disconnected figures, strong dark outlines. "It reminds me of broken pieces being put together," I commented.

Jim pointed to the picture and then deliberately patted his hand on his lap.

"Is that how you feel?" I asked.

Jim pointed to his ears.

"Broken hearing?" I asked.

He shook his head, said no aloud and pointed higher.

"Broken mind?"

He nodded.

It was an exquisitely painful and beautiful conversation. Jim felt that he was in shards. A weight seemed to lift when he found a way to tell me so. On follow-up visits, we explored the image more and because Jim is a person of faith, we talked about where God is in our brokenness, how God might be in the seams of the pieces, where the vibrant colour in life is in spite of the awkward piecing.

We engaged the art and let it inform our spirit. We weren't afraid to make mistakes. In fact, there were no mistakes to be made. There was no need to improve anything. The creative exercise was all about entering into what was already there.

The sky is the limit when it comes to caring through creativity. There are boundless forms to explore: visual arts, music, drama, dance, writing, and crafts such as knitting and pottery. Check out Gary Glazner's Alzheimer's Poetry Project (APP),[19] Judith Friedman's Songwriting Works,[20] and Elizabeth Lokon's Opening Minds through Art.[21] These are all wonderfully inspiring programs and resources designed to engage creativity. Best of all, they are beautifully suited for those who have dementia and their caregivers.

Whatever the artistic medium you are exploring with your loved one, let curiosity be your guide. Ask questions, wonder aloud, and collaborate. Sharing a creative experience can enhance your relationship. You might be surprised at what emerges.

When I invited Joe to dance in a sacred movement session, his wife Nancy piped in, "Joe never liked dancing." Undeterred, I stretched out my hand. "Do you want to dance, Joe?" I asked. He took my hand. We proceeded to sway holding hands in time to one of Joe's favourite hymns, "Will Your Anchor Hold?" For the first time in his life, Joe was liturgical dancing and having a great time doing it. Nancy was gobsmacked. Dementia removed Joe's inhibitions and he discovered new loves, including waltzing in the living room with Nancy. She too discovered that she could cut a rug. A new dimension of their relationship opened up.

Potential lies at the heart of creativity. When we tap into our creativity, we often discover new possibilities.

Artist Willem de Kooning continued to paint long after his diagnosis of Alzheimer's. His style became more free form and colours more vibrant later in the disease process.[22] Similarly, French composer Maurice Ravel wrote *Boléro* in 1927 after some researchers say he started to experience symptoms of dementia.[23]

Above my office at the church, Chris White runs a music group for people with dementia and their caregivers. I swear when the group gathers, the hallways sing. The upbeat energy is palpable. White's care is inspiring. Beyond leading group activities, White has made albums with participants. Once, he rented a nearby theatre where people with dementia and their caregivers did musical performances.

"We put too much emphasis on language," he once told me. "The brain might not have semantic ability anymore. So what? That brain might still be capable of learning new things. We've got other channels, like rhythm, laughter, and just being in the group together to explore ... This is a creative adventure. We are creating with dementia. We're not just babysitting or going gently into that good night. We are going with a big noise."

The great religious studies scholar Thomas Merton (1915–1968) once wrote, "Art enables us to find ourselves and lose ourselves at the same time."[24] When we are creative, we lose our anxiety, our stress, our loneliness. We find connection, peace, and a deeper sense of self. Great reasons to tap into fresh, creative ways to express care!

If you aren't sure where to start, try one of these 50 ways.

1. Read a favourite poem. Contemplate words and phrases that have meaning.
2. Cut beautiful images out of magazines, newspapers, etc., and make a mosaic.
3. Take in a virtual art gallery tour.
4. Attend a concert.
5. Try simply moving to different styles of music.
6. Go for a walk and intentionally notice the colours and/or sounds.
7. Plant flowers, fruits, or vegetables.
8. Compile a playlist of favourite songs.
9. Make a centrepiece.
10. Cut out random words and piece them into a poem.
11. Experiment with ways that music can boost mood – play tranquil music when you sense anxiety, happier music when feeling low in energy.

12. Make sculptures out of clay.

13. Create installations with miniature objects that hold meaning.

14. Turn an ordinary lunch into a picnic.

15. Admire the work of a famous artist or composer. Discuss what you like about it.

16. Go outdoors and make a found-art installation with twigs, leaves, rocks, etc.

17. Take photographs and turn them into a calendar to share.

18. Using watercolours, practice making brushstrokes in time with music.

19. Colour in an adult colouring book.

20. Find items around the house that have texture. Make prints with them.

21. Explore chair yoga.

22. Draw action words out of a hat and improvise movement.

23. Conclude story starters like "Once upon a time ..." with words or actions.

24. Doodle.

25. Get a variety of paint swatches. Ask, "Which colour most appeals to you? Which colours calm you? Which ones make you feel happy?" Make a collage based on the colour. Frame it so you can revisit it.

26. Experiment with coloured chalk on a chalkboard.

27. Put wet paint in the centre of a piece of paper. Fold the paper in half. Open it and discuss what the image reminds you of.

28. Pick foliage and flowers to arrange.

29. Create cards and mail them to friends.

30. Pour brownie ingredients into a jar and drop it off to a neighbour.

31. Admire the view from a window, noticing the shapes and shadows of things.

32. Find percussion "instruments" around the house and play along to a song with a good beat.

33. Look at favourite photographs. Discuss what's in the foreground, background, how it makes you feel, etc.

34. Bake something yummy.

35. Draw or paint your emotions.

36. Keep a journal for a specific period of time using words and/or images. Look back from time to time. What do you notice?

37. Draw a perfect day.

38. Consider a number of quotes. Frame a favourite one.

39. Create a collage from images that make you happy. Give it a prominent home.

40. Put images of things you value most into a jar. Give the jar to family and invite them to add to it.

41. Paint a rock. Add a message to it. Place it somewhere it can be found.

42. Build a personal altar. Include in it images that you feel blessed by.

43. Pick a colour and take a walk. Notice everything that is that colour.

44. Look at nature paintings. What do you like best? Practice making your own.

45. Create a memory box of items that have particular meaning. Consider taking photographs of each item and sharing an album with family.

46. Make wind chimes out of shells and other found objects.

47. Compile interesting textured fabrics. Make a collage. Which ones are most attractive?

48. Reconfigure a variety of shapes cut out of paper to make as many creations as possible.

49. Sing along to favourite songs.

50. Make paper flowers and give them away.

SCRIPTURE: GENESIS 2:4b–7

In the day that the Lord God made the earth and the heavens, when no plant of the field was yet in the earth and no herb of the field had yet sprung up — for the Lord God had not caused it to rain upon the earth, and there was no one to till the ground; but a stream would rise from the earth, and water the whole face of the ground — then the Lord God formed man from the dust of the ground, and breathed into his nostrils the breath of life; and the man became a living being.

QUESTIONS FOR REFLECTION AND DISCUSSION

1. In what ways are you creative and how are you caring creatively now?

2. Are there other creative avenues you could explore to support you in caring?

3. Where do you sense God's creative spirit at work in your caregiving?
4. What aspects of God's creation do you find most wondrous? How can you connect more with them?

SPIRITUAL PRACTICE: *VISIO DIVINA*

Visio divina has been practiced since the early Middle Ages. The Latin word *visio* has to do with seeing and *divina* refers to what's divine. So *visio divina* is a way of seeing through God's eyes. The spiritual practice is based on the idea that God is everywhere and present in everything and is a way of interacting with an image, a piece of art, or something we see in the world around us.

1. Find an image that speaks to you. The image might be a painting at home, a photo in a magazine, a sculpture, or simply what you see when you look out the window.
2. Notice the image. Consider the colour, texture, mood, style.
3. Slow your breathing.
4. Gaze at the image. Focus. Let your eyes soften. If your attention wanders, bring it back to the image. Engage your imagination to enter the image and explore it. Notice every aspect.
5. Ask, "Where am I most drawn to this image? How might divine love be expressing itself through this attraction?"
6. Listen to how God is speaking to you through the image.
7. Give thanks. Express gratitude to the creator, who has blessed you and who is drawing you to new ways to love creatively.

SPIRITUAL PRACTICE: POETRY MEDITATION

1. Choose a poem that speaks to you.
2. Underline the words that resonate.
3. Wonder, "What is it about the ideas I've underlined that speak to me? Why am I drawn to those ideas at this point in my life journey? Where is the Spirit nudging me through those ideas?"
4. Meditate/dwell in gratitude for the gift of the spirit.

PRAYER

Let's not go gently into that good night.

Let's go creatively.

Let's go beating our own drums and singing our own songs.

Let's go dancing with great, awkward, and elegant exuberance.

Let's go leaving wild marks only understandable to us.

Let's go with luscious tastes on our tongue.

Let's go with rich earth embedded in our nails.

Let's go with montages of hope filling every space.

Let's go with soul-stirring colour and scintillating texture.

Let's go creatively.

For we are – all of us – going,

but we are not yet gone.

Go with us, God.

Amen.

7

Facing Giant Moments

"Alzheimer's may steal my mind over the next few years,
but I am not going to let it steal my joy in the years
leading up to it. I can't control what is going to happen
to my brain, but I definitely can control how I handle
the situation for as long as I can."
– Kelly Bone, *in her blog*
Living My Best Life with Alzheimer's

Six cubits and a span. In other words, over nine feet tall. That's how big the Bible says Goliath, a member of the Philistine army, was.

David's brothers were already doing battle with Goliath when David's father seconded him to take food to the battlefield. On his way there, he heard stories of the giant and how fearful the Israelite army was of him. He asked King Saul to let him take a shot at defeating the giant.

Maybe the young upstart's bravado impressed the king. Whatever the case, Saul sent for him. When David insisted on fighting Goliath, Saul laughed. "You are just a boy, and he has been a warrior from his youth" he said.

"Your servant has killed both lions and bears; and this Philistine shall be like one of them," David argued.

The next thing he knew, David was staring up at Goliath across the field. He retreated to a brook nearby and chose five, smooth stones. He put them in his pocket and set off to confront the giant. All nine feet of him.

You know the rest of the story.

But did you know that the tallest person in recorded history is a fellow by the name of Robert Wadlow who stood eight feet, 11 inches tall?[25] Inches shorter than the biblical giant.

A Goliath seems humanly impossible. That's the point. The story is about confronting something bigger than you can fathom, something so imposing, so looming that it shadows you.

And that's possible. As caregivers, we stand in the shadow of feelings, decisions, and questions all the time. We can find ourselves in such weighty, overwhelming moments that any move we make feels crushingly wrong. Often, we land in these moments when the personality of the person we are caring for changes.

Dementia can affect personality and behaviour. Sometimes these behaviours are hard to manage and so we label them "challenging." Without a doubt, some behaviours can be challenging to us as caregivers. They can feel like Goliath issues, even when we know that they are not intentional.

Thinking about these behaviours less as challenges and more as expressions of emotions or ways of communicating might help us respond more effectively. Sometimes the biggest Goliaths, especially during a frustrating day, aren't the behaviours that the person with dementia we are caring for is exhibiting but our response to them.

Elizabeth sank into the chair in my office, physically drained and overcome with guilt. She is her mother's primary caregiver. "A couple of hours ago, I lost it," she explains. "It happened when I tried to get her in the shower." Initially, Elizabeth tried to coax her mother into the shower, telling her she would feel better when she finished. When her mother resisted, she attempted to reason with her. "I told her she could get sick," she said. Next, she tried to physically pull her mother toward the bathroom. When her mother refused, Elizabeth yelled at her: "Why do you always have to make everything so hard?" and stormed out of the room in a torrent of colourful expletives.

"I feel so terrible. Do you think I'm a terrible person?" she asked.

"I highly doubt anyone as dedicated to their mother as you are is a bad person," I responded.

The conversation turned to why her mother resists showering. "Maybe because it's so intimate? Maybe the water is too cold or hot? Are depth perception issues making the bathtub seem scary? Is she exerting control in areas of her life that she can?"

We decided that instead of worrying about getting her mother to shower, Elizabeth would focus her energy over the next couple of weeks trying to figure out why she didn't want to. A month later, she showed up at my office door looking visibly relieved.

She had presented her mother with choices, inquiring if she would like her to help with the shower or if she wanted Elizabeth to hire someone. Her mother chose the professional. "She's always been a private person," Elizabeth reflected. "She goes along with Alice [the homecare worker]. I think maybe she doesn't want us bathing her."

Sometimes the Goliaths aren't the way that those we love are expressing themselves. Sometimes our approach to caring is the giant we need to overcome.

Offering choices can afford those we are caring for a sense of control and agency over their own lives. Arguing with a person who has dementia or trying to persuade them by outlining facts is often futile. If the person can't follow the logic or remember from one moment to the next or just plain doesn't think what you are suggesting is in their own best interest, there is little likelihood of success.

Alzheimer's associations recommend strategies such as reframing and refocusing. Turn orders like "Get off the couch!" into invitations: "Let's go make dinner." Instead of instructing "Come and help clean this up," express what you need: "I could really use your help cleaning up. Can you help me out here?"

Consider the sticky situations you face. Would changing your approach help? Brainstorm strategies. Dementia support groups and societies have loads of advice and suggestions about fresh approaches to try when challenges loom large. No matter the advice, determining the best response to the common experiences I outline below ultimately rests on our ability to discern well. Hold your dilemmas, whatever they may be, before God. Pray for wisdom and insight.

When David went down to the water to choose stones for his sling, he picked up five. Why five? I think David was coming up with a contingency plan. Maybe he would miss. Maybe another Goliath would step up. David was realistic. There will always be Goliaths. There will always be challenges.

The truth is that there will always be problems that are nine feet tall. That's the bad news.

But the Christian story, the faith story, is about good news. There will always be solutions. Maybe one. Maybe five. That means there will always be opportunities to give it your best shot. We're not going to hit the target every day. But we aren't at a loss. Our hope doesn't lie in what we can't solve; it lies in what we *can* solve. It lies in the resources we can pull together to take our best shot. Trying our best is the best we can do.

Here are some tips to help.

Coping with aggressive speech and actions

Remember that those who say hurtful things or act out aggressively do not intend harm and they aren't to blame. Dementia experts say that it's best to view the behaviour as an attempt to communicate a need, want, or desire. According to the Alzheimer's Society of Calgary, it's best to avoid arguments and confrontations. Validate and respond to the emotion instead of the content of what the person has said. Say "I hear that you are upset. I'm so sorry you are feeling that way. I'm here with you and want to help."[26]

Medications can have side effects. Before turning to them, try to identify when the problem arises and discern the level of danger it poses to your loved one and others.[27]

Take note of when the person is most aggressive. Do you notice any patterns? If you do, can you make adjustments? If, for example, your loved one expresses themselves aggressively at mealtime, changing the seating arrangement or the food itself could reduce stress. If sundown is difficult, playing soothing music or using aromatherapy may bring calm. Any unexplained changes of behaviour warrant a visit to the doctor.

Limiting wandering

Six out of ten people with dementia wander.[28] Although it may seem pointless, wandering often has a purpose. Is wandering in the night triggered by a toileting need? Would posting bathroom signage on the door or installing a nightlight help? Is daytime wandering caused by boredom? What would happen if more activities were scheduled?[29]

Although it can be good exercise, wandering can also be hazardous. Remove throw rugs and wayward cords to prevent falls. When you go out, stick to the same route and avoid busy roadways to reduce the likelihood that people with dementia will get hurt or lost if they venture out.

Is it time to think about making physical changes to doors? If so, the National Institute of Aging based in the United States suggests keeping the door locked and installing bolts on the highest or lowest point of the door so long as there is an emergency exit plan in place. They also suggest posting a prominent stop sign; keeping shoes, purses, and other signs of departure out of sight; installing a device that signals when a door or window opens; and placing removable gates, curtains, or bright streamers across the door.[30]

"It can be expensive, but putting up a fence – with secured gates – can stop wandering while giving your loved one a way to get some fresh air," suggests WebMD, adding that radio tracking devices can also be helpful. "Bracelets or other jewelry with radio transmitters can be a big help. Some are short-range and designed so that caregivers can keep watch on the person themselves. Some sound an alarm on both the bracelet and a base unit when the person gets too far away."[31]

Preventative measures such as sewing an address into a coat, putting location devices in shoes, or purchasing an ID bracelet with your contact information engraved on it can increase the likelihood that your loved one will be found if they get lost. Consider giving your friends, neighbours, and local business owners your contact information. Develop an emergency folder for backup. Include your address, a current photo, names and nicknames that your loved one responds to as well as a list of places they like to visit.

Responding to "I want to go home"

Home is where the heart is. We know from experience that home is more than a roof over our heads and a place to sleep. When a loved one with dementia says they want to go home, what they might actually be saying is that they long for what home represents: safety, comfort, and belonging. "'Home' may represent memories of a time or place that was comfortable and secure and where they felt relaxed and happy. It could also be an indefinable place that may not physically exist," advises the Alzheimer's Society.[32] It's best not to correct or dissuade them from wanting to go home.

Instead, be attentive to when they ask to go home. Are there particular patterns? Do they ask for home at a certain time of day, during a particular activity, or only inquire with one person? Can you change any of these situations to be more peaceful? Use a redirect strategy. Begin an activity that is enjoyable to take your loved one's mind off wanting to go home. In some cases, talking about home can be comforting. The award-winning caregiving website *Daily Caring* suggests inviting conversation. "Asking about their home validates their feelings, encourages them to share positive memories, and distracts them from their original goal of going home. Open questions that encourage them to share their thoughts work well. For example: 'Your home sounds lovely, tell me more about it. What's the first thing you're going to do when you get home? What is your favorite room of the house?'" [33] Reassure your loved one that they are safe and that people care for them right where they are.

Answering queries about a person who has died

Sometimes it's hard to know when to tell the truth and when the truth will cause harm. The best response depends on the stage of dementia as well as your loved one's frame of mind in the moment.

Pay attention to the feeling behind the longing. Like homes, people can represent safety and comfort. When someone we love dies, we miss how we feel when we are with them: safe, comforted, happy. Validate feelings. Try saying, "It sounds like you miss XYZ very much ... tell me about them." Diverting attention from grief by inviting the person to join you for a walk or another activity can sometimes be helpful.

In her book *Surviving Alzheimer's: Practical Tips and Soul-Saving Wisdom for Caregivers,* Paula Spencer Scott suggests trying a variety of approaches, including gently orienting our loved one to the reality of death and then reminiscing: "'Wasn't she the sweetest person ever?' 'I'll always miss her piano playing. I remember the time she gave that concert at the school ...' Don't make a big deal about insisting the person absorb the reality. There's no need to drive him to a cemetery to 'prove' the death or show an obituary, for example. Logic is ineffective," says Scott. [34]

If it's best in your case to share the reality that the person your loved one is seeking has died, be sure to confirm they aren't in pain. Occasionally, people with dementia will have full conversations with the person who died, believing that they are still present. If these chats bring comfort, they are a blessing.

Broaching the inability to drive

Raising the topic of no longer driving is one of the most sensitive and grief-laden issues that caregivers confront. It's best to get ahead of the decision. Discuss the subject in the early stages of dementia so that the person you care for can be involved in making the decision when to stop. Decide at what point symptomatically the person feels that they should no longer get behind the wheel. Consider signing a driving contract (ask the Alzheimer's Association for a sample to get you started) that names who your loved one wants to tell them when it is no longer safe to drive, giving them permission to take measures to prevent them from getting behind the wheel.[35]

The goal of care is always to support independence. The Alzheimer's Society of Canada suggests that while symptoms are mild, steps can be taken to help loved ones drive safely, including settling into a consistent routine, sticking to the same route, driving with someone, and using assistive devices such as a GPS. When safety becomes an issue, empathize with your loved one's grief. Ask them how they feel. Don't correct. Reassure your loved one that as painful as it is, life goes on after driving. Work with them to decide which form of alternative transportation would work best – public transit, taxi service, family, friends? If the discussion becomes difficult, a clinical assessment can help people with dementia gauge when it's no longer safe to drive.[36]

Addressing inappropriate sexual behaviours

Sexuality is part of being human. The desire for intimacy doesn't go away just because a person's brain isn't firing correctly. Inappropriate sexual behaviours like making lewd comments, self-pleasuring in public, and pursuing intimate relationships can be distressing for caregivers. Ask yourself, is the sexual expression harmful? If it's appropriate to the relationship, maybe it's best not to worry. Would more frequent hugs or caring touches help? If hypersexuality is directed toward a caregiver who is not a spouse, see if a different caregiver has an impact. Making clothing modifications can be helpful or putting a pillow or fidget board in a person's lap might make a difference.

There may be other reasons for the behaviour. For example, attempts to remove clothing could be a signal that the person is too hot or the fabric is bothersome. "Acts like public undressing or genital touching may be misinterpreted as sexual, when in fact they can result from pain, discomfort, hyperthermia, or attempts to be freed from a restrained environment," write Drs. Riccardo Di Giorgi and Hugh Series. Don't be embarrassed. Indifference to sex and inappropriate sexual behaviour are common symptoms. Discuss your concerns with a doctor so that you can determine the appropriate next steps.[37]

Encountering a reluctance to bathe, eat, or take medication

No caregiver wants to force the person they are caring for to bathe, eat, or take medication when they don't want to. But not looking after them properly can be neglectful and dangerous.

Experts suggest first trying to discern where the resistance is coming from. Does the person dislike the food, or are they no longer able to

see it? Are they scared of the water or embarrassed? Are they reject-
ing medication because they no longer recognize and therefor trust
the person giving it to them? Sometimes knowing the "why" behind
the person's resistance can lead to creative solutions.

Try offering choice: apple or banana? bath or shower? take the pill
with lunch or dinner? Enhancements and incentives can help. "Dad, I
bought your favourite cologne. Smell it. It's great. After your bath, we're
going to put it on." Or, "We're going to go the doctor now and afterward, we are going to go to Louis Restaurant. We'll split a pepperoni
pizza. Their sauce is so good."

The Mayo Clinic suggests explaining your needs, presenting a trial
run, and describing care positively. "Don't ask your loved one to make
a final decision ... a trial run will give a hesitant loved one a chance to
test the waters and experience the benefits of assistance ... Refer to
respite care as an activity your loved one likes. Talk about a home care
provider as a friend. You might also call elder care a club or refer to
your loved one as a volunteer or helper at the center."[38]

Remind yourself that the person is unwell and not wilfully trying to
be difficult. Consider changing your expectations. It might not be okay
to skip the medication but perhaps delaying the bath for another day
isn't the end of the world. If the situation gets stressful, take a break.
Circle back when everyone is calm.

Dealing with delusions and paranoia

In the mid to later stages of dementia, delusions can become problem-
atic for the caregiver and frightening for the person with dementia.
Your loved one may believe a family member is trying to poison them,

so they refuse to take their medication. Or a friend is trying to steal something, so they hide their belongings.

This can be shocking, especially if the accusations are levelled at you. Remember that this is a symptom of cognitive decline and not intentional. What's more, the person with dementia may be truly distressed. Seek medical evaluation to rule out any other causes for the delusions like an infection or a negative drug interaction. If your loved one is being cared for by others, maybe their things truly are going missing. Keep an eye out.

The golden rules of other scenarios apply here too: Don't argue. Stay calm and state the truth. Distract and redirect. "Switch the focus to another activity. Engage the individual in an activity, or ask for help with a chore," says the Alzheimer's Association. "Duplicate any lost items. If the person is often searching for a specific item, have several available. For example, if the individual is always looking for his or her wallet, purchase two of the same kind."[39]

Try mirroring your loved one's feelings and restate your caregiving purpose. "I can see you are worried, Mom. I'm sorry you feel that way. I'm here to help."

Deciding to let go of some caregiving responsibility

Discerning when to seek additional caregiving support, whether by engaging outsiders – family, friends, or professionals – or placing our loved one into continuing care requires knowing what our loved one wishes, and/or self-awareness on our own part. Ask clarifying questions: Are either you or your loved one unsafe? What is your stress level? The Alzheimer's Association *Caregiver Stress Check*[40] can help you determine if your stress level is overwhelming. Are you letting things slide that affect your health and well-being, such as cleaning your home, paying bills, and taking care of personal hygiene? These are all potential signs that change is required.

Consider in-home care, respite care, or a housing situation where there is additional support. Dementia societies can help you identify possibilities. If you and your loved one decide that they need to move to a continuing care centre, these same groups can give you tips to find the right one, prepare for the move, and adjust to the new living situation.

For some of us, letting go of or sharing responsibility can be excruciating. We can be reluctant to share caregiving tasks because we feel that in some way we have failed our loved one. Talk to someone who has been where you are, who knows the grief, guilt, and relief that you might feel.

Know that seeking help doesn't mean that you don't care. Quite the opposite! As long as our loved one is alive, we will continue to care. The type of caregiving role we play and the tasks involved, however, may change. Whatever decisions you make, remember that your loving, caring role will remain as important as it ever was.

Assuming decision-making power

In earlier stages of dementia, people with dementia can develop a decision-making plan, including preparing for long-term care and health interventions, making financial arrangements, and naming persons to make decisions. In later stages, it can be harder to determine when to step in. Your local Alzheimer society or association has valuable information about substitute decision-making for health care and finances, advance directives, and competency assessments. They can also give you tips and advice about if, when, and how to intervene. Seek out their help.

Remember that supporting the independence and autonomy of the person you are caring for is always the goal. That means including the person with dementia in decision making as much as possible. Just because they may not be able to make some complex decisions doesn't mean your loved one is not able to make *any* decisions. Also, the capacity to make decisions can fluctuate. Schedule critical conversations at the best time for the person you care for. Offer prompts or cues to help make the decision at hand. If they can't make the decision, put yourself in their shoes. What would they do? Consult others (family and friends) who know the person to confirm that the decision you have made is the right one. Always put the person's best interest first.

SCRIPTURE: 1 SAMUEL 17:40

Then he took his staff in his hand, and chose five smooth stones from the wadi, and put them in his shepherd's bag, in the pouch; his sling was in his hand, and he drew near to the Philistine.

QUESTIONS FOR DISCUSSION AND REFLECTION

1. My biggest caregiving giants are ...
2. I could face them better if ...
3. I feel most accomplished as a caregiver when ...
4. Come what may, I trust that God will ...

SPIRITUAL PRACTICE:
MORNING/EVENING PRAYER MOVEMENT

Dance and movement were common features of Christianity until the 16th-century Reformation when liturgy became more focused on words. Today, Christian groups are recovering the idea that we can worship God not just through our words but through our whole being. Less wordy and more embodied ways of worshipping are important, especially as we look for fresh ways to explore spirituality with people with dementia. In the morning or evening, do this gentle moving prayer as many times as it feels good, either seated or standing, alone or with the person you are caring for.

God, I'll praise you in the morning. *(Slowly raise your arms from your sides over your head.)*

I'll praise you in the evening. *(Stretch your outstretched arms up to the sky and "twinkle" your fingers.)*

I'll praise you in my sleeping. *(Gently do a side bend, stretching from one side and then the other.)*

I'll praise you in my living. *(Place your hand on your heart.)*

Repeat.

PRAYER

The sky's the limit with you, Holy One.

I wish it were so for me, too.

But I'm human to the bone,

so very human.

Help me accept my humanity with all of my limitations and potential.

When I'm inclined to dwell on dilemmas, wrongs, and "can'ts"

ground me in your spirit.

Remind me I'm not you and that's okay.

Turn me toward hope.

Raise my spirit to soar alongside you.

Show me what's possible.

Help me see through your eyes.

Amen.

8

Making You a Priority

"Anne will burn out. I'm afraid.
I don't like it. Not me. Tell her I'm next.
Second. She's important."
– Bruce

The rains came. It rained and rained. Noah kept sending out a dove, praying that the nightmare would end soon. Still, for 40 days, there was nothing (Genesis 7:17). Forty is a symbolic number in the Bible. It represents infinity. So for what felt like an eternity, the rains came.

Fast forward. Everyone survived. The animals lived to see the rainbow. Noah and his family lived long enough to get off the ark.

They weren't exactly skipping off it, though.

The only thing harder than building the ark might have been getting off it.

The ark delivered Noah to a world he didn't know anymore. The landscape he had known his whole life was gone. There were no trees. The ground was a wet mess. And there was no one left to talk to but his family who was on the boat with him.

He knew how to build an ark because God gave him all the specifications. God told him to make it from cypress and to create rooms in it. Leave space between the roof and the opening. Make three decks. Construct a door.

But there was nothing now that the rains stopped. No instructions. No idea what to do first or next. How to live. Because there was no normal. There were no roads to follow. No signposts. No rules. No structure. What Noah saw when he stepped off the boat was emptiness. A world of emptiness.

The story continues that Noah planted a vineyard. One day, he erected a tent, got drunk and passed out naked. One of his boys covered him up. He woke up cursing (Genesis 9:21–28). And then the story reports that he died.

Some people blame Satan for the intoxicating properties of Noah's wine. I think Noah knew what he was getting himself into when he had a drink. I think he was exhausted. Burnt out. He'd do anything to make it stop.

In his drunken state, he curses his son, Canaan. Logically, it made no sense but Noah was worn out. Who can blame him?

We have all lashed out from time to time, typically when we are at our lowest point. Noah's story is assurance that we are not alone. Even the most capable people have their moments. The great patriarch charged with saving the world wound up getting drunk, falling naked into a tent, and waking up cursing. These punishing words are the last ones the Bible records Noah saying before he dies.

It's a cautionary tale. We can take care of the whole universe but if we don't take care of ourselves, we will wind up in a sorry state.

Caregiving can feel as exhausting, exciting, and purposeful as building an ark. It can feel like we're adrift forever. It can feel like intimate connection with God, and like endless chores and an exercise in perseverance. It can feel like getting off the ark, too, with all the disorientation and rebuilding that entails.

The more caregiving responsibilities we have, the more likely we are to feel the weight of our role. Some of us present an "I got this" attitude to our families while in reality we are a breath away from dropping.

That's where Sara was when she stopped by my office. Every fibre of her being screamed exhaustion when she plunked down across from me. When I asked how she was doing, she told me about how her sister Betty was increasingly forgetful and resistant.

Betty could no longer help with the kitchen duties and had started to wander such that Sara felt she always needed to be within sight.

"How are *you* doing?" I asked again.

She rhymed off a list of shoulds: I should be more together; I should have more patience; I should be more motivated.

"Sara, I notice that when I asked how you are doing, you told me about Betty and when I asked again about you, you shared a list of what you should be doing. If you were sitting in my chair, what would you say to yourself?" I asked gently.

She started to cry. "I don't know."

We've all been there. So in tune with the needs of the person we are caring for that we set our own care needs aside. If we don't sacrifice ourselves, we feel selfish, indulgent. We know the classic argument about self-care: if we don't care for ourselves, we won't be able to care for our loved one. It seems well and good in theory but when we are really in the thick of caregiving, it can feel completely unrealistic. Who has the time and luxury?

Self-care as a concept is applied to everything from taking a bubble bath to lighting aromatherapy candles. At its heart, though, self-care means tending to mind, body, and spirit. It's about making the most compassionate choices in all areas of life, including making caring choices for ourselves. We don't practice self-care solely so that we can care *better*, as if we are a means to an end, but because *we, like everyone else, are worthy of care.*

Caring for ourselves is pretty countercultural. That's why we have a hard time doing it.

Until the 1960s, self-care was a medical idea. It had to do with enhancing health and preventing disease. With the rise of the women's and civil rights movements, self-care was reframed as a political act, a way of taking control over your own body rather than allowing sexist medical practices to stake a claim on it.[41]

Although the idea has gone more mainstream, self-care remains subversive. Especially for caregivers.

We are socialized to give caregiving our all, even ourselves. The more we sacrifice, the more we care. The more we give, the more virtuous we are. So we prioritize ourselves last. In so doing, we can become depressed and burnt out.

Are you losing interest in relationships and activities? Do you find it hard to get to sleep, stay asleep, or wake up? Are you getting sick more often? Do you struggle with feelings of hopelessness, irritability, and forgetfulness? Are you self-medicating with drugs, alcohol, or abusing sleep medication? Do you feel that caregiving is all-consuming?

These can all be signs of burnout and compassion fatigue. If you are experiencing these signs, seek out support. Talk to your family doctor. Confide in a friend.

Finding support does not mean that you are a failure. Caregiving can be really hard. You are not alone.

Caregiver burnout has been described as "a debilitating psychological condition brought about by unrelieved stress."[42] Do you feel constantly stressed? Are you sending out a proverbial dove day after day like Noah did, hoping for any positive sign that you may be able to get off the caregiving boat soon?

Did you know that in Canada, 33 percent of senior caregivers describe the caregiving experience as stressful or very stressful?[43] According to the Anxiety & Depression Association of America, between 40 percent and 70 percent of family caregivers show symptoms of depression "with approximately a quarter to half of these caregivers meeting the diagnostic criteria for major depression."[44]

"The expectation that we can be immersed in suffering and loss daily and not be touched by it is as unrealistic as expecting to be able to walk through water without getting wet," writes Rachel Naomi Remen in *Kitchen Table Wisdom: Stories That Heal.*[45]

Caregiver stress can lead to burnout and ultimately to compassion fatigue. Unlike slowly burning out, caregivers suffering from compassion fatigue can quickly find themselves losing empathy for those they are caring for, and unable to refuel.

Sara had many of the high-risk factors for caregiver stress. She was living with her sister full time, had suffered depression in the past, didn't feel that she had a choice in becoming a caregiver, and spent most of her day playing caregiving roles. There were no other family members left and she felt alone. By the time she sought me out, she was showing signs of compassion fatigue. She had begun not to care about Betty, even resenting her.

"I lost it when she refused to put on her shoes. I yelled at her and knocked over the plant," she said, her voice laced with shame. "I'm not myself," she whispered.

In some cases, caregivers can become abusive. Sara clearly needed to take a step back. We worked to arrange respite care, began to put in place self-care strategies, and made an appointment to speak to a psychiatrist. In the end, Sara found the balance she needed to care well for both her sister and herself.

The best way to prevent caregiver burnout and compassion fatigue is to get in front of it. Fortunately, there are tips and strategies we can put in place to help.

Do a self-care review

In what ways do you take care of yourself? That's not a rhetorical question. Count the ways. Write them down. Which ways of caring for yourself make you feel the best? Are there old ways of caring for yourself in the past that worked and/or new ways that are worth a shot? How many minutes or hours do you spend each week caring for yourself? How much time do you think you need? How can you take one more step toward getting what you need? What might need to change in your life to carve a path of self-care? What resources are available to you to make that change?

Put on the lens of compassion

Do you need to direct compassion toward yourself? No matter what you feel (sad, exhausted, angry, grateful, loved, etc.), compassion begins with acknowledging that your feelings are valid. Other care providers have experienced what you are experiencing, including one of the Bible's greatest heroes. Enough with the judgment! Instead of beating yourself up, dive into those feelings and uncover lies beneath them. Do you feel trapped or unappreciated? If so, what would make you feel less stuck and more appreciated? Maybe you feel sad. What specific part of your situation makes you feel most sad? What would make your sadness more bearable? Imagine Jesus is sitting across from you, speaking words of compassion. What is he saying? Let your heart absorb his words.

Pay attention to your self-talk

Our self-talk can take a toll on our ability to cope and to thrive. Whether we are consciously aware of it or not, we are always interpreting the circumstances we find ourselves in, filtering them through a complex system of experiences, assumptions, and worldviews. It is one thing to label a particular caregiving experience difficult. It's another to say, "This is hard because I am a lousy failure." Sometimes we don't even realize the scripts we repeatedly play in our mind. Carry a notepad with you for a day. Write down every negative thought. Review your script. What do you notice? Repeat the exercise. Are there patterns? Try changing the script and see what happens. Replace "I hate doing this" with a question: "What is one thing I can do to enjoy this task more?" Would playing a favourite tune while performing a caregiving task you don't enjoy help? Would providing an incentive when you complete the task – maybe a bath or an hour with a good book or favourite program – help you face it? What messages do you most need to hear? Perhaps you are making signs and instructions for your loved one with dementia, hanging them as prompts. What signs could you create for *you*?

Take a break

I know what you're thinking: there aren't enough hours in the day; if you don't "do," no one will and then what? Yet you also know that even machines break down and that if you treat yourself like one you won't be at your best. Worse, you might wind up like Noah – passed out in a tent and cursing the wrong people. If you can't arrange respite, hire or invite someone to help. Several organizations for caregivers advise working micro-breaks into your schedule. Take five minutes to meditate, watch a video, flake out on the couch, stretch, or write. Try to schedule more five-minute breaks or work to stretch them into ten minutes. If you only have a minute, pray the one-minute prayer at the end of Chapter 4.

Let go of perfection

I hate to break it to you, but ... you aren't perfect. Actually, none of us are. Our caregiving will never be perfect either. We aren't always at our best. Instead of focusing on setting the bar higher, focus on what you are able to give in the moment, and on the spirit with which you are offering care. Congratulate yourself often. One caregiver I know left affirmations around the house: "You rock!" "You are enough!" and

"Doing my best is the best I can do." To maintain perspective, take stock of your successes. Note the countless ways your care makes a positive difference in the life of the one you are caring for. Maybe the person with dementia is no longer able to express their thanks. Imagine what they would say if they could express gratitude to you.

Control what you can

Preparation is key to feeling in control. Have your affairs in order (draft a legal will, establish power of attorney for care and financial matters, etc.). Get organized. Keep lists of medications, routines, and appointments, to help provide structure, and to establish and stick to routines. Eliminate clutter in your surroundings. Tackle the junk drawer or the overstuffed closet. Just by adding structure and simplicity in your life, you can free up energy for what's most important.

Connect with others

We can get so hunkered down into our caregiving role that we find ourselves isolated and detached from the world around us. Connecting with others is a core human need. When we don't feel connected, we can become depressed, moody, and even more stressed. Ideally, we can schedule time to go out to meet with friends and family, or with a support group. If that isn't possible, a phone call usually is. Just chatting with a neighbour can brighten the day. If you have access to the Internet, find a few minutes to connect online. Intellectually, we know that we need to connect. In fact, we know we need to eat well, reach out, and take a break, too; where the rubber hits the road is how we plan to do it.

Reach out for help

Similarly, we need to reach out for help. Let go of "keep a stiff upper lip" and "pull yourself up by your bootstraps" thinking. Humans aren't designed to go it alone. We were born to be in relationship with one another. In his classic book, *7 Habits of Highly Effective People*, Stephen Covey writes that the goal of life isn't independence; it's interdependence.[46] Interdependence means we rely on each other but aren't controlled by the other. In times of stress, we can be tempted to hunker down and withdraw into ourselves. It's those very moments when we are tempted to retreat, however, that we most need companionship and care. Reach out. Don't shoulder your care in isolation. Instead, think about ways you might be able to build and tap into a team of caregivers.

Assemble a team

Several Alzheimer's Associations recommend assembling a team, advising people with dementia and caregivers to reflect on the skills of family and friends. Do any of your family or friends have the time and skills to help with specific tasks, such as grocery shopping, or to give you an hour of down time? Are there dementia societies in your neighbourhood that have support groups or resources that can help? Is your family doctor helping you to come up with a strong care plan? Do you have a good attorney and financial planner? Are there other caregivers on- or offline that could help you brainstorm scenarios, or with whom you could compare notes about your daily experience? Can your faith community, or pastor, lend support? Are private caregiving services available? Consider all of these human resources as your team and invite their support. Know that you aren't imposing. All of us want our lives to have meaning and purpose – you are giving someone the opportunity to use their best skills and abilities to make a difference.

Care for your body

Eating well and getting enough sleep and exercise are a self-care nobrainer. But it's easier said than done. Days can blur into weeks or months and we suddenly realize that our only form of exercise is rambling to the kitchen, our drink of choice is anything caffeinated, and we've eaten whole meals out of the cookie jar. Instead of trying to turn yourself into the paragon of fitness overnight, make small changes. Just eight to ten minutes of exercise here and there adds up. Top your cereal with fruit to amp up the nutritional content. Replace one cup of coffee or can of soft drink with water (add ice and lemon or get fancy by adding frozen berries if it helps) to reduce energy crashes. See your doctor for a checkup. Make sure you keep all your medical appointments. "There is no royal road to anything. One thing at a time, all things in succession. That which grows fast, withers as rapidly. That which grows slowly, endures," is widely attributed to American novelist and poet Josiah Gilbert Holland. It's simple advice. Don't worry about taking on the big picture, just take the next small step.

Nurture your spirit

Caregiving is an extension of the heart and therefore, by definition, a spiritual exercise. Studies show that caregivers who don't practice spirituality are more stressed and anxious. Family caregivers in particular report high levels of spiritual distress. Nurturing your spirit is core to your well-being. Is there a spiritual leader or community that can be a source of strength for you? What spiritual practices most resonate? I've included several meditations, affirmations, and prayers in this book. Try them out. If you discover one through which you feel connected with God, with something larger than yourself, lean into it. Search out additional similar practices and make space in your life for them.

Dwell on what's good

Our thoughts can be our best friend or worst enemy, and sometimes the hamster wheel in our brain gets the best of us. Focusing on everything that's going wrong can prevent us from seeing what's going right. It's important to look critically at ourselves and at our circumstance, but it's equally important not to dwell on the things we can't control. When you are in a mental rut, intentionally switch your thoughts. Consider what's possible. Think about all the things you have learned and accomplished. Give yourself a gold star for everything you are doing. Express gratitude, even and especially for the little things. Know that you are making a difference through your care.

SCRIPTURE: JOHN 10:9–10

I am the gate. Whoever enters by me will be saved, and will come in and go out and find pasture. The thief comes only to steal and kill and destroy. I came that they may have life, and have it abundantly.

QUESTIONS FOR REFLECTION AND DISCUSSION

1. How does caring for yourself contribute to abundant life?
2. Name things that diminish your capacity to have abundant life. What can you do about them?
3. Noah went through life phases: building the ark, enduring the storm, rebuilding. Do any of these resonate with you?
4. What does, or could, "abundant life" look like in the phase of life you are in?

SPIRITUAL PRACTICE: LISTING ABUNDANT LIFE

Never underestimate the power of the humble list. For well over 2,000 years, faithful people have been making lists to stay focused, remember, and prioritize. The Ten Commandments is essentially a list of to-do's, and there are many tongue-twisting genealogical lists scattered throughout the Bible. This spiritual practice invites you to turn a humble list into a meaningful guide toward living an abundant life.

1. Make a list of things that contribute to your sense of well-being. It could include things such as exercise, quality time with family, recreation in nature, a good night sleep ...
2. Beside each of these things, write why you want them. For example, I want to exercise so that I have more energy. Dig deeper. Reflect on why you want what you want. For example, I want to have more energy so that I feel better when I give care.
3. Spend some time in prayer, listening to where the spirit is drawing your attention. Considering all the things you have

named that lend to your well-being, where is your attention drawn? How might God, divine love, be expressing itself in that attraction?

4. Underline the aspects you feel called or urged to prioritize.

5. Ask for God's support to help you prioritize those aspects.

6. Decide to do one thing this week, no matter how small, that will help you take the next step toward making this thing a priority.

7. Thank God for being with you in this time of discernment. Pray for strength, wisdom, and insight to take the next steps to care for yourself.

A LIST OF COMMITMENTS TO CARE FOR MYSELF

1. I will do my best and my best today may not be my best yesterday or tomorrow.

2. I will be open to blessed moments.

3. I will care with dignity and respect.

4. I will regard myself with compassion.

5. I will intentionally seek joy.

6. I will remember to feed my spirit.

7. I will treat my body with care.

8. I will recognize but not dwell on negative thoughts.

9. I will trust in my gifts and abilities.

10. I will let go of things beyond my control and trust in the power of God to uphold and guide me.

May it be so, O God. Amen.

9

Tending
to the Spirit

"I am mad at God. I also feel like I have so much good in life.
Is it selfish to be frustrated? I wonder where God is
or even if there is one.
I don't know if I should say that."
– Gerald

Apparently, God is fond of road trips. The Bible tells stories about how God's people traipse through deserts, climb mountains, and venture across lakes, fields, and cities. It shouldn't be a surprise, then, that instead of telling Jeremiah outright what he should be prophesying, God sends him on a field trip.

"Go down to the potter's house," God says. "There I will let you hear my words."

Sigh. Jeremiah heads to the studio. He hangs around, waiting on God. It feels like hours. Still, no message. Bored, he watches the potter work. Clay whips off the wheel. The potter retrieves it, presses it into a new mound and begins to spin it yet again, his fingers boring into the centre.

Then, Jeremiah hears the voice of God: "Can I not do with you just as this potter has done? Just like the clay in the potter's hand, so are you in my hand ..."

Jeremiah is being worked on. Worked through. That's the message.

Don't we all need to hear that the hand of God is always upon us, shaping and re-shaping our spirit? It's good to know that even when we feel unqualified, God is present, caring through us, the potter's hands shaping us all the while.

As humans, we are deeply spiritual. That means as caregivers we have a built-in knowledge of how to care for our loved one's spirit.

Religious or not, we are all well-acquainted with spiritual needs: the need for hope, for belonging, for love, and for meaning. All of us are qualified to offer spiritually oriented care. Spiritual care is vital, especially given that the systems we are immediately thrust into when we become ill have such a profound impact on our spiritual well-being.

Unfortunately, when we are sick, our experience is heavily mediated through a medical model of care. As soon as we become ill, we enter a medical system that defines us as a "patient." We learn to talk medicalese, sharing our experience of illness through the lens of treating and curing. The system is a product of and contributes to what psychologist and author Arthur Frank calls Western culture's restitution narrative of illness, which positions us to anticipate getting well again and as such makes curing the goal. The narrative goes like this: I am sick. I was healthy. I will be well again.[47]

Where does that leave our loved ones with dementia who have no hope of becoming as healthy as they once were?

On one hand, they are told to want and strive for restoration; on the other hand, they are advised to accept decline. Inevitably, they wind up stuck.

As caregivers, we can free our loved ones from this narrative by encouraging them to tell a more fulsome story of their experience of living with dementia. An experience that involves love and loss, pain and joy, alienation and companionship.

That's where spirituality comes in. The spiritual quest for meaning is about the soul's restoration, achievable to our very last breath.

I was ordained as a United Church minister in my early 20s. At that point, I hadn't experienced life-limiting illness and hadn't endured the deep losses that I have become well-acquainted with since. My idea of death was entirely negative. It was something to be feared and staved off. It didn't occur to me that illness and even pending death can actually be the rich earth that spirituality roots in, the fertile ground from which meaning springs.

Then I met my friend Ruth, a palliative care nurse. I commented that it must be hard to do her job, to be around suffering all the time.

"Well, no. The opposite," she said. "That's exactly the time when the spirit can truly soar."

Through illness, suffering and loss, she taught me, there is a deepening capacity to ground our spirit in what matters most. That doesn't mean we have to like it, but it does mean that we can draw nearer to God in the midst of it.

Over the years, I've come to understand that my role as a caregiver is to accompany people on a journey into what is most meaningful and life-giving. I have had the deep privilege of witnessing the spirit take root in the most challenging circumstances. I can't count the number of times I've sat at someone's bedside and heard them say in a voice tinged with irony, "Here I am dying and I've never felt more alive."

Judy never finds my responses to her existential questions completely satisfying. "You never answer my question," she complains as she reformulates the same question she has asked me many times before: "Is there a God and why would God make me go through this?"

"I believe that God is the impulse to love that flows through the universe," I repeat. "But God's ways are mysterious. None of us will ever know the mind of God. I don't think God creates suffering, but I definitely think God is present in it. Tell me about how you are suffering."

Judy's eyes wince as she begins to share. A minute later, they fill with tears. When she finishes, her shoulders have visibly released. I pray, lifting to God all of Judy's questions and suffering, asking for courage, strength, and the insight to witness the presence of love in her life. Afterward, we are silent for a moment.

"Judy," I ask gently, "where do you experience love in the midst of your suffering? I think that's where God is."

Caring for a person's spirit isn't simply about promoting a particular religious practice such as prayer (unless it's helpful) or one belief over another; it's about being present to another's spirit and being open to and wrestling with existential questions such as Judy's, most of which none of us have "answers" for.

Frankly, I don't know the reason why there is suffering in a person's life or in any of our lives for that matter. I don't see it as my job to speculate or to offer ready answers. My work is to be attentive to why a person is asking the questions.

I think of spirituality as the quest for wholeness, for meaning and purpose. It has to do with those deep questions all of us ask, especially when we are confronted by our own vulnerability and limitations: Why has this happened to me? Is there life after death? Who am I now? What's the point of it all? What can I hope for?

It's important as caregivers to listen, not to respond, but in order to bear witness to another's heart. When it comes right down to it, few of us have people in our lives who are *able* to hear, much less who *want* to hear, about our suffering. Even when they do, sometimes we shield them. I don't know about you, but from time to time I avoid talking about the things that pain me so that my loved ones don't suffer.

Listening to – witnessing – someone's suffering is a tremendous, sacred gift. In fact, it's one of the most meaningful gifts we as caregivers are perfectly positioned to offer because it means that our loved ones don't have to bear their pain alone.

"How are you doing today?" is not a question of convention or a passing sentiment. When we care for the spirit, we truly want to hear the response, as difficult and pain filled as it may be.

Offering spiritual care isn't for the faint of heart. It's much easier to dispense a pill than to bear witness to pain or to hold space for someone's grief. It's also easier to slide into dispensing advice than to listen with an open heart.

Holding space for hard feelings is, well, hard. It's good to call in a higher power.

Before I enter any hospital room to care for a family, I pause to pray. I ask God to be present in me and to give me wisdom and insight that my care might be in some way healing. When I walk through the door, I know that I am not alone.

When you find caring for the spirit hard, pause and say a prayer. Being present to suffering and grief isn't always easy because most of us have a lifetime of experience trying to avoid it.

Our culture teaches us that pain, suffering, illness, and grief are entirely bad. It encourages us to applaud people who are ill for their courage or positive outlook while they are sick. I think that's because, collectively, we are uncomfortable with feeling out of control.

We talk about "battling" and "beating" illness so that we feel we are in the driver's seat. The problem with framing illness that way is that those who die are seen as losers because they have lost the battle. It also means that anyone with a debilitating, life-threatening illness or condition are automatic losers because they are doomed upon diagnosis. The language of conquering illness and of maintaining positivity heaps pressure on people who are ill to deny what they are feeling, leaving them alone when they most need support.

Avoid the instinct to comfort by offering words that prevent people from honestly sharing. "You will be okay," for example, might sound soothing but may actually prevent the person who is ill from saying that they are *not* okay.

Don't worry – talking about fear, pain, and loss doesn't make it worse; *not* talking about it does.

Providing strong spiritual care means not only being a companion on life's beautiful peaks but also in its devastating valleys, accompanying people through the grand vistas and the frightening caverns. When we as caregivers hold space for suffering, pain is drawn into healing light.

True healing takes more forms than fixing bodies. Sometimes healing looks like the restoration of relationships, or release from shame, or the capacity to forgive and let go, or the courage to go on.

So where do we start, especially when not all of us are comfortable talking about matters of the spirit?

Do you fear that your communication might segue into tensions over religion, or that you might seem intrusive or awkward, or get caught in theological conversation that you aren't equipped for? Remember, your role even when you are intentionally caring for the spirit is not to have all the answers or to register a religious opinion; it is to witness the experience of the person you are caring for so that they might find meaning and purpose in their lives. In this venue, a good question is much better than a quick answer.

Start by asking if this is a good time to have a meaningful conversation. It might sound strange, but asking permission means that the person you are caring for is in control.

Spirit-oriented questions such as "What's important to you?" and "What brings meaning/strength/comfort to you at this time?" can launch a sacred conversation.

Try using "mirroring" techniques to empathize. Paraphrase what the person has said so they feel heard and understood: "It sounds like you are in pain because you feel dementia is removing the control you once had over your life. Am I right about that?" Extend the offer to share more deeply: "Tell me more about what that's like for you."

Medical doctor and author Eric Cassell says that suffering occurs when a person feels that their sense of self is threatened and that it continues until the threat passes or the person establishes a new sense of self in the face of it.[48] Active listening helps people to articulate who they are in the midst of suffering and to move through it to a renewed meaning and sense of self. Finding meaning, strength, and connection is the antidote to spiritual distress.

That's why it's so important not to brush off pain.

The saying "God never gives us more than we can handle," for example, can shut down the person's desire to share whereas the question "Do you feel that some days you have more than you can handle? ... Tell me more about that ... " is an invitation.

Similarly, saying "God lets us suffer to teach us a lesson" suggests that the root of suffering is God and that the point of the suffering is growth. Sure, illness can move us to grow, to be more compassionate, and to advocate, but what kind of God needs to cause us to suffer to do that? Surely, God could think of more positive ways to teach us a lesson? It might be better to ask, "How has your experience of suffering had an impact on your spirit?"

As caregivers, it's crucial that we are real in the moment. Don't guarantee a miracle cure or tell your loved one that their health will improve if you are pretty sure it won't. Instead, focus on what you can guarantee: care that maintains dignity, pain relief, the fact that you will be there every step of the way, that they are loved, God's spirit is always present ...

In the story from Jeremiah, God uses few words. Instead, the writer uses the metaphor of a potter sculpting clay to get the message across. The things of the spirit can help us care, especially if language is an issue. In fact, the objects that we surround ourselves with have spiritual significance, whether we are conscious of it or not.

I visited Gary's apartment not long after his wife died. He was chronically ill and always felt that his illness held him back from doing what he loved. I noticed that every single piece of artwork on his wall depicted a home in a rural setting with a fence across the front, the gate always closed. "Gary, have you ever noticed that all of your beautiful prints feature a closed gate?" I asked. Unconsciously, he was expressing his frustration in his surroundings. It was an epiphany. I wondered aloud what would help open the gate. The art became an intentional tool for spiritual reflection. Eventually, as he identified the closed gates in his life and began to consider ways to open them, Gary replaced all of his paintings with new pictures of open gates!

David Morgan, an expert in visual religious culture, once told me during a recorded interview that images have emotional impact because of their effect on the brain. Similar to what happens in the brain when we hear music, "When we see things, we code them in several different ways. We code them in terms of memory. We code them in terms of rational thinking. We code them linguistically. We code them emotionally. These structures of the brain are enmeshed. Images are powerful because they stimulate these various brain centres, integrating the systems," he says. That's why the "stuff" of spirituality and religion can remain recognizable even in later stages of dementia.

When I offer care in the dementia unit of a nearby continuing care centre and don't know a person's spiritual or religious background, I bring a box filled with religious objects. There's a cross, rosary, menorah, and statue of Shiva as well as things that are more spiritual than religious-oriented, such as a rainbow, a candle, a rock, and a peace symbol. I carefully show these to people and invite them to choose one that has meaning to them. I wonder aloud about what they have chosen and then play a song or say a poem or prayer associated with it. The objects very often facilitate relationship and sharing. Along with music, prayer, and meditation, I consider them spiritual caregiving resources.

Think about the things that your loved one surrounds themselves with. Through them, can you foster connection? Could you work any of these into a routine or ritual?

Wilma's family told me that throughout her life Wilma was an avid atheist, but she didn't mind when I visited her. The first time we met I opened my box of spiritual things and showed them to her. She gingerly took out the battery-operated candle. Eventually, I lit it at the end of each of our visits. When I did, we took a moment to be thankful for family and friends, and to hope for good things for them and for Wilma herself. It became our little ritual.

Rituals like going to worship, saying grace, or lighting a candle can be grounding. Does the person you are caring for have any spiritual rituals? Can they be more intentional or even enhanced? Could you take a few more seconds over grace to light a candle? Can an evening prayer or playing a spiritual song or meditation be a welcome addition to your caring routine? Would hanging a cross or a photo that holds deep spiritual meaning in a prominent place be comforting?

Caring for the spirit well means being intentional about our words, our space, and our rituals, but, mostly, caring well means listening with our whole heart. Never underestimate what just being present means.

You don't need to have all the answers or the right words or the right objects or rituals. None of us ever do. Call on the spirit to guide your loving intentions. You'll get where you need to go.

SCRIPTURE: JEREMIAH 18:1–6

The word that came to Jeremiah from the Lord: "Come, go down to the potter's house, and there I will let you hear my words." So I went down to the potter's house, and there he was working at his wheel. The vessel he was making of clay was spoiled in the potter's hand, and he reworked it into another vessel, as seemed good to him. Then the word of the Lord came to me: Can I not do with you, O house of Israel, just as this potter has done? says the Lord. Just like the clay in the potter's hand, so are you in my hand, O house of Israel.

QUESTIONS FOR REFLECTION AND DISCUSSION

1. How do you intentionally offer spiritual care? If you don't, what's preventing you?
2. Have you ever had a "potter's house" experience? When have you felt like you were sent on a divinely inspired field trip?
3. Jeremiah gained insight into the reality of his relationship to God through experience as much as or more than through words. How does this have meaning for us as we care for people with dementia?
4. When has just having someone listen been a gift to you?

SPIRITUAL PRACTICE: SILENT MEDITATION

Noise is a constant in our world today, as are communications. Silence is one of the ways we break free from the hustle and bustle of our to-do's and from the should-do's that roll around in our minds. Silence is a discipline that helps us discern the voice of God more clearly. Make this meditation as short or as long as you need it to be.

1. Take slow, deep breaths. Inhale through your nose and exhale through your mouth. Pay attention to your breathing.

2. Release the chatter of your mind. Let unwanted thoughts go and focus on your breath. If your mind wanders, bring it back to your breath.

3. Begin to notice the presence of the holy. Sometimes it's helpful to visualize this as a light or as a heart.

4. Open your heart to hope, peace, joy, and love. Just "be" in the presence of God.

5. Relax and enjoy sacred presence.

6. Close with a prayer of gratitude.

PRAYER

Caregiving God,

on my best days, you celebrate with me.

On my mediocre days, you point me to gratitude.

On my worst days, you carry me.

Morning to night you shape my life with meaning,

restoring me even as I sleep.

Thank you,

my carer,

my confidant,

my friend,

my creator,

for all the ways you impress my life with your spirit.

Amen.

10

Talking to Children

"I want my grandchildren to know that I love them.
That's the hardest thing – to think about not
being able to tell them. I'm writing letters to each one
now so that if I get to a point where I can't tell them,
they'll be able to read the letters for themselves."
– Ruth

The guest musician sits on a stool in the centre of the family room of a long-term care facility, animatedly playing and singing "The Hokey Pokey." At his feet, preschoolers are excitedly doing the actions. Around the perimeter, elders and staff smile brightly as they watch the children dance and sing. Three seats down from me, an elderly gentleman stares at his hands, his head hunched over his chest not appearing to be engaged in the singsong.

Nearby, one of the children stares at him with a curious expression on her face. She becomes too preoccupied with the man to follow the musician. I watch her walk over to him, reach into her pocket, withdraw a piece of paper, and hold it out. When he doesn't reach out to take it, she picks up his hand and places the paper in his palm. It is a crayon drawing of a sun. The little girl could have picked any one of the 40 or so people in the room to give her drawing to, but I sense she knew who needed it most.

Children have love to give.

No wonder Elijah envisions a small child leading the Israelites to restoration. Later, Jesus, indignant that the disciples were sending away children, said, "whoever does not receive the kingdom of God as a little child will never enter it" (Luke 18: 16). In other words, transforming and amazing grace is expressed and achieved by the least powerful and most insightful. Both Elijah and Jesus teach that children are our spiritual teachers. They aren't becoming deeply spiritual – they already *are* deeply spiritual.

That's why children are terrific caregivers. Those who have been raised with empathy are naturally inclined to express love. As much as we want to protect them from life's difficulties, experience with diverse people fosters compassion. A child's-eye view of the world can be a refreshing, educational balm for us as caregivers, too.

Here are tips to help you speak to the children in your life about dementia.

Share the diagnosis

"I don't want to tell Natalia about her grandfather's dementia. I don't want to scare her," her mother Rose told me. "But then I also want her to be able to visit and understand what's going on. What should I do?" she asked.

Rose's question is a common one. We instinctively want to shield our children. But honestly is the best policy. Children are inherently perceptive beings, sensing feelings in the air.

"It can be reassuring for children and young people to understand what the problem is. If they are not told the truth about what is happening sooner, they may find it difficult to trust what someone close to them says later on. It may also be more upsetting for the child or young person to find out about a diagnosis later than to cope with the reality of what is happening now," advises the UK based Alzheimer's Society.[49]

Find a good time for a conversation when there aren't a lot of distractions. Consider this the first of several discussions.

"Think about your child's developmental stage. Younger children aren't going to be able to understand or handle very much, whereas an adolescent can understand much more and will want and need to know much more," writes Dr. Claire McCarthy in an article published by Harvard Health Publishing. "Younger children can be very concrete and might worry not only that they can catch the illness, but also that it's their fault. Older children can understand more nuance and complexity and will have very different worries."[50]

The age of the child and the closeness of their physical and emotional relationship with the person who has dementia will have an impact on what and how you share the diagnosis with them.

Toddlers, for example, don't have an understanding of illness or a disease process. They are much more likely to process what's happening intuitively and be more attuned to your energy. A calm, non-anxious presence will speak louder than words with these little ones.

Some time after two years of age, children begin to understand illness. But even then, before divulging the diagnosis, it's good to get a sense of their level of awareness. Draw out their understanding by asking if they have noticed Grandpa or Aunty doing something that feels different. Their astuteness might surprise you. You might even tell them so.

Gently but matter of factly explain that their loved one has been diagnosed with dementia, a condition that affects the brain. Emphasize that the child didn't cause it, can't catch it, and that it is something that mostly affects older people. Be reassuring but honest. If you don't know the answer to a question, say so and offer to try to find it.

Explain biological processes in age-appropriate ways

Explain biological processes as simply as possible and expand your explanation as the child asks more questions. The Alzheimer Society of Canada's "Just for Kids" information sheet begins this way: "Dementia affects the person's brain. There are some diseases that cause the brain to stop working properly, and you may start noticing some changes in the person who has dementia. When people have dementia, they may forget, they may get confused, they may have trouble speaking and taking care of themselves."[51]

Some children will want to know more about how the brain works. Show a picture. Explain that the brain is in charge of our thoughts and behaviours. Different parts of the brain have different responsibilities. One part is responsible for how much we remember. Another, for how we move. When a person has dementia, parts of the brain become damaged and start to die. If the cells die in certain parts of the brain, people behave differently.

Resources tailored to your child's age/stage can help you find the best way to share information. Alzheimer's Research UK's web page Dementia Explained[52] offers a wealth of age-appropriate information to help explain dementia to young children, juniors, and teens. Dementia Australia's website, Dementia in My Family, also offers sound tips and advice.[53] Check out *The Dragon Story* on YouTube, a short cartoon for five- to nine-year-olds, that explains dementia and how it can affect family members.[54]

Tell them what they can expect

Once the child has an understanding of the illness, move to what they can expect to experience. Explain that as brain cells die, more parts of the person's memory will be affected.

Ask the child what their pet's name is or the name of the street they live on. How did they remember that? Explain that their brain allows them to remember important information. When a person has dementia, they might forget their name, the words for things, or even what they just said. They might get lost easily and find it hard to do the things they used to do.

Here's how the Alzheimer's Association's "Parent's Guide" suggests honestly answering a child's question about their loved one's prognosis: "Your uncle will have both good and bad days. Even though there are no treatments or a cure yet, scientists are working really hard to find them."[55] Your child might also benefit from understanding the biological progression: Dementia gets worse over time as more brain cells are affected.

Honour feelings, no matter what they are

Whatever the child is feeling, acknowledge it. They may feel angry and upset that their loved one has a disease and that their life might change as a result, or they may feel annoyed that they have to hear the same story repeatedly. It's okay if they tell you that they feel bored or embarrassed when they visit their loved one.

Explain that their feelings are valid and help them to find healthy ways to express them. Share what you do with your feelings: How do you express your sadness? What do you do when you feel angry? What do you try to focus on when you are bored or embarrassed? Talk to them about what they have done in the past with their hardest feelings. How did working through those feelings help?

Empathy and role-playing

Empathy, the ability to understand and feel the emotions of another, is something children develop over time as their brains mature, but there are activities that can help them develop this ability with someone who has dementia. Play music from a number of competing sources at once to help your child understand why some people who have developed sensitivity to sound find it hard to concentrate with background noise. Invite the child to pull a cap down part way over their eyes as they navigate the living room to illustrate why they need to draw closer to a person whose vision has been impacted by dementia.

The Alzheimer's Society's "Dementia Resource Suite for Schools" suggests a number of different awareness building activities: "What's Missing?" involves covering objects with a blanket, removing one, withdrawing the blanket and asking the children to identify what's missing. Gradually, as more objects are added, the game gets trickier. Afterward, ask students questions: Why is this activity difficult? What makes it harder? How do you think people who have difficulty remembering things would cope with this activity? What does our memory do? How does it help us in our lives?[56]

Role-playing can also help develop empathy. If they are old enough, invite your youngster to assume the role of the person with dementia and you become them. Play out a typical interaction. Ask the child what they notice it's like for the person to have dementia and invite them to coach you on what they need.

Reflecting on a situation that you have experienced with the child and asking questions can help build empathy: "It's natural to feel frustrated with Nana when she can't remember our name. When I feel frustrated, I try to imagine how I would feel if I was Nana. How would you feel if you couldn't remember your best friend's name? How would you want to be treated if you forgot?"

Studies show that one of the best ways to foster empathy is to consider what we have in common with another person. Invite the child to think of the things they have in common with Papa. Maybe they both enjoy chocolate or ice cream. Maybe they like music or going outside. Stress that all of us know what it means to feel loved and that people with dementia always know when they are loved.

While we might be tempted to reward children for their caregiving efforts, incentivizing a visit with a new toy or money may backfire in the long run. Instead, boost the child's self-esteem by emphasizing the positive qualities in the child that are evident when they are visiting.

Remember you are a role model

One day, I told my four-year-old son we were going to do dishes together. I pulled the kitchen chair up to the sink and began to fill it with water. "Wait!" he yelled and scrambled off the chair. He went and got the phone, wedging it between his shoulder and pressing it to his ear. "Ready now!" he declared. It turns out he wanted to do the dishes "like Mom," who as he observantly emulated, is the queen of multi-tasking.

Brain research has uncovered unique cells called mirror neurons. When we observe, we activate mirror neurons that forge the same neural connections made from doing the behaviour ourselves. In other words, we are wired to learn through observation.

Whether we are doing the dishes or caregiving, the children in our midst are taking their behavioural cues from us. Children are like sponges, learning how to give care by watching our techniques. Be intentional about what you want them to learn. Actions speak louder than words!

Offer reassurance in difficult moments

Children sometimes blame themselves when an interaction with a person with dementia is confusing or difficult. Experts advise clearly explaining that problems in the brain are causing the way the person with dementia is expressing themselves. Let them know that the person with dementia loves them the same as they always did, but can't control what they do or express their love the way they would want to.

If the child is confused by the words a loved one is using, make sure they know that the person believes they are using the right words. Make a game of talking to your child with your lips closed like a ventriloquist. Guess what each other is saying. Explain that persons with dementia know what they are saying but sometimes have a hard time finding the right words. That's why it's really important we find ways without words to show that we care.

Avoid overloading responsibility and focus on growth

Giving children a role in caregiving is important but it's possible to overdo it. Be sure that caregiving activities don't absorb time from friends, hobbies, homework, and other kid stuff. Offering an appropriate level of care can build compassion, empathy, self-esteem, creativity, and resilience. Invite your child to think about how caring for their loved one helps them to grow as a person. Connect them with caregivers their own age. "It's fun seeing her. We chat a lot. I take her for walks. We sit in the lounge. It's good to see her. I feel like she remembers me sometimes in the things I do," says Dan, a young person featured in a video he filmed for Alzheimer's Research UK: *Dementia Explained.* "It's a lot of responsibility because I feel that I've got to take care of her and it's kind of hard. I manage with it. It sets me up for life. You just gotta go with it. She's still with us, just in a different way."[57]

Brainstorm ways to love

Children naturally have love to give. They are wonderfully creative, too. Invite them to dream up ways to show love with and without words. If they are drawing a blank, explore possibilities: invite them to share a piece of music, an album, or to bake something special. They could create a memory book and include stories of themselves when they were little spending time with the person with dementia and some of their best memories together. Offer conversation topic prompts for the next visit: friends, hobbies, sports, school ... place all the topics in a jar and have fun discussing them one by one at the next visit. There's no limit on love. Have fun finding fresh ways to express it together.

SCRIPTURE: MARK 10:13–16

People were bringing little children to him in order that he might touch them; and the disciples spoke sternly to them. But when Jesus saw this, he was indignant and said to them, "Let the little children come to me; do not stop them; for it is to such as these that the kingdom of God belongs. Truly I tell you, whoever does not receive the kingdom of God as a little child will never enter it." And he took them up in his arms, laid his hands on them, and blessed them.

QUESTIONS FOR REFLECTION AND DISCUSSION

1. What do the children in your life teach you about caring?
2. How do you model caring?
3. What do you think Jesus meant when he said that we need to receive the kingdom of God as a little child?
4. What child-like qualities would it be helpful to have?

SPIRITUAL PRACTICE: SACRED DANCE OF GRATITUDE

Children are beautifully expressive, especially with their bodies. They are unafraid and unashamed to move, to dance. Put on a favourite

music and they rarely sit still. Try ripping a page from their playbook!
Dance like no one is looking.

1. Play a favourite piece of music that makes you feel good to be
    alive.
2. Begin to move to it, feeling the rhythm and beat, swaying to the
    melody.
3. Focus on feeling free and open.
4. Begin to note what you are grateful for. As you move, name
    people and pets that enrich your life. Give thanks for mentors,
    confidants, providers. For the loyal spirits, the generous ones,
    the loving ones.
5. Give thanks for kind acts, for warm smiles, for the beauty of
    nature.
6. As you dance, feel gratitude welling up and uplifting your spirit.
7. When the music concludes, notice the feelings of your body and
    breathe. Rest quietly. Note how you feel now compared to how
    you did before you danced. Sense God's blessing in all the things
    you expressed gratitude for.
8. Give thanks for the dance of beauty and blessings in your life.

PRAYER

Wrap my care with the wisdom of youth, O God.

Enfold me in childlike spontaneity.

Cover me in curiosity.

Warm me with imagination and energy.

Calm me to be truly present in the moment.

Wrap your arm around me.

Stay a while.

Read me the story of your great love,

again and again.

Amen.

11
Widening Circles of Care

"I want to do what I always have. Go to the gym.
The hardware store. It's not so easy anymore.
I get flustered. It's embarrassing.
Sometimes I just leave or don't go at all."
– Andrew

Jesus ate a lot. He invited himself over to Zaccheus' house for dinner, fed 5,000 people on a hill, advised his followers to invite strangers to dinner, dined with his closest friends on the eve of his death, prayed for daily bread, and was frequently accused of eating with "tax collectors and sinners." After his resurrection, his disciples didn't recognize him until he broke bread with them.

Jesus wasn't just being hospitable or forging relationships across the table; he was breaking boundaries. In the culture of his time, who you ate with, what you ate, and how you ate it reflected the tightly controlled social order. You weren't supposed to eat with people of a lower social class, for example. When food was served, the most important guests were served first and ate the best. That's why Jesus ruffled feathers when he said things like, "When you give a luncheon or a dinner, do not invite your friends or your brothers or your relatives or rich neighbours ... invite the poor, the crippled, the lame and the blind." He also said things like, "When you are invited by someone to a wedding banquet, do not sit down at the place of honour ..." The table became such a subversive cornerstone of Jesus' ministry that theologian Robert Karris says he got himself killed by the way he ate.[58]

In the Christian tradition, no matter your denomination, a central sacrament is Communion or the Eucharist. Sharing the holy supper is one way we express Jesus' subversive hope for a world where everyone is welcome at the table, a world where we care enough about one another to extend the invitation.

Humans beings aren't designed to care alone. We are called to be caregivers for one another. As much as the rampant individualism prized by Western society tries to convince us otherwise, we know we care better when we feel well supported, when there are others we can count on to care, and when community and organizational leaders think of themselves as caregivers.

"The delusion [of individualism] is a kind of prison for us, restricting us to our personal desires and to affection for a few persons near us," Albert Einstein once wrote in a letter to a rabbi. "Our task must be to free ourselves from this prison by widening our circles of compassion to embrace all living creatures and the whole of nature in its beauty."[59]

How would your life as a caregiver change if the responsibility of caring belonged to everyone? If our collective social goal was to widen circles of compassion? What would it mean to the persons we care for to know that every social circle – every table – would not only welcome them but value their contributions?

For 75 years, psychiatrist Robert Waldinger and his team of researchers followed 724 people to learn about what constitutes a "good" life. His findings boil down to what we know through experience – good relationships are key to both happiness and health.[60]

Too often, I've heard friends with dementia and caregivers tell me that the condition itself doesn't cause them as much suffering as social exclusion does. For these people, watching friends fall away and avenues for participating in society slowly dissipate is painful. Loneliness hurts emotionally and physically. Among other things, it affects brain health. When we are lonely, studies show we process information more slowly, perform worse on tests, and are more likely to be anxious and depressed. In turn, our ability to think suffers. Not only does social exclusion exacerbate dementia, but recent research says that it is causes a 50 percent increased risk of it.[61]

Dementia societies, caregiver associations, and informal networks are doing wonderful advocacy work to support caregivers and those we care for. Our fellow caregivers who have fewer caregiving responsibilities often provide valuable insight and advocacy in the public arena for those who have more. Still, there is more work to do and, unfortunately, sometimes as individual caregivers we find ourselves in situations where we have to advocate for ourselves. The words to express our own needs and desires don't always come easily.

I've written this chapter not so much to convince you that circles of care need to be widened – I'm sure you are acutely aware of that! – but to share some words and ideas to help you advocate for what you and your loved one need.

Here's a running list of tips and advice I share with community groups seeking to widen their circle of care. It is by no means extensive, but it may give you a starting place to flesh out a list uniquely tailored to your circumstances.

Become more informed

In the world's largest dementia-related stigma survey, two-thirds of the nearly 70,000 people who responded think that dementia is a natural part of aging.[62] The idea that dementia only happens to older people is one of many myths about the condition.

Knowledge leads to empathy and understanding. The first step is becoming informed. Dementia associations and societies have a wealth of information about types of dementia, symptoms, and strategies to not only include but benefit from the capabilities of persons with the condition. Learn about dementia first-hand from people you know. If you are in a position of leadership in a school, business, or religious organization, run an awareness program, bring in a speaker or invite people to share their experiences of living with dementia if they are open to doing so.

Foster belonging

Belonging is one of the most fundamental human needs – and among the oldest. Our ancestors needed to belong to kin groups for safety and survival. Belonging continues to be central to our physical, mental, and emotional well-being. Basic respectful manners can go a long way toward fostering belonging. Don't talk over, correct, test, or ignore persons with dementia. Check out blogs, books, and other resources created by people with dementia to express their experience living with the condition. Simply passing along first-hand accounts of living with dementia on social media and in friend groups can contribute to the culture shift that needs to happen so that people feel heard. In the last decade, Memory Cafés where people who experience memory loss and their caregivers can socialize and enjoy activities have cropped up all over the world. Initiatives like these strive not only to offer stimulation and respite but also a sense of togetherness. Communities need to host more of these safe spaces where people are not reminded of limitations or judged for behavioural differences, and where everyone is free to join in or not as they wish.

Know the risks and take action

Lack of awareness of dementia and its symptoms not only leaves people isolated, it's life-threatening. For example, 60 percent of people with Alzheimer's will wander and up to half of those who do will suffer a serious injury or death if they aren't found within 24 hours. People with dementia may not remember their name or seek help when they are lost. Simply asking someone if they are lost and need help can save their life. Sometimes the person will be carrying an alert system such as a bracelet, or have an address sewn into their jacket, or be carrying identification in their wallet. If you can't find identifying information or are uncomfortable inquiring, contact the authorities and stay with the person until they arrive. Don't worry about being intrusive; better safe than sorry! Imagine if their primary caregiver is fran-tically looking for them. More broadly, communities can choose proactively to implement public notification systems such Silver Alert,[63] to help find missing persons with dementia.

Be an open presence

Most of us take for granted being able to do the essentials: buy grocer-ies, get our hair cut, visit the bank, order a sandwich at a restaurant, and so on. But each of these things can present challenges for loved ones with dementia and the more stressed they are the more challeng-ing daily tasks can become. One survey revealed that 69 percent of people with dementia said the main reason they stop going out in pub-lic is lack of confidence. Being a helpful, unhurried, calm presence can make an enormous difference. Don't underestimate the power of say-ing hello and asking someone about their day. Simple exchanges can mean the world. Just offering to help, indicating that there is no hurry, making eye contact, and being friendly and open are simple ways eve-ryone can embody compassion and care.[64]

Go beyond welcome and inclusion

It was 11 o'clock on Wednesday and I answered a knock on the church door to find Mary standing with her hands on her hips, angry that the church was closed. "You can't have service without me," she huffed. Startled, it took me a few moments to realize Mary thought it was Sun-day. We sat down in the empty sanctuary and said the Lord's Prayer after which I walked Mary home. It was the first of many mid-week knocks on the church door and angry protests.

Clearly, dementia diminished Mary's capacity to know the date and time, but it didn't reduce her desire to be faithful or to be an integral part of the community. Recognizing her longing to be included, church members started picking up Mary for services and individual members began to go to the local coffee shop with her. Her family lived over seven hours away and the church filled a kinship role that much of the time she was missing.

Mary also offered her talent to the church, filling envelopes, helping with events and children's activities. She was well-cared-for by our community but we also benefitted from her presence.

The problem with a vision of welcome and inclusivity is that someone is always doing the including, usually the person or persons who have the power to. What's more, inclusivity can be based on sympathy or duty rather than on the recognition that everyone has something to offer. As communities, we are stronger together. Work toward becoming more than friendly and inclusive. Acknowledge everyone's contribution. Celebrate difference. Let people know you value their presence.

Create opportunities to contribute

Dementia-friendly activities can bring joy and foster connection. But we need to do more than pass time to feel fulfilled; we need a sense of purpose. My grandmother who is 93 years young and coping with memory loss finds meaning knitting to raise money for a program dedicated to helping first responders. While she attends craft groups where she lives, it is most fulfilling for her to contribute to her community. Before my mother retired from teaching, she facilitated reading outings to local continuing care centres. The students would read to seniors, some of whom had dementia. In return, the seniors acted as mentors. A win-win!

People with dementia are a wonderful, untapped resource for communities, which can benefit from their time and talent. Imagine the difference it would make to a struggling coffee shop that might gladly alter the atmosphere (dim lights, quiet music ...) to enjoy more patronage; or to a non-profit struggling to do a mailing if they had volunteers to help. The possibilities for real contribution are endless; intentionally let those with dementia know what they can do to help.

Support people with dementia and their caregivers in the workplace. Solid staff are the most valuable resource in any workplace. Some workers who develop dementia while employed avoid disclosing their diagnosis, fearing stigma and reprisal. Unfortunately, this means a delay in putting proper supports in place that would relieve stress, improve productivity, ensure that the employer can benefit from expertise as long as possible, and mitigate errors. Foster an open workplace culture. Learn about how many employees are impacted by dementia and caring responsibilities by circulating a survey. Publicize workplace issues that caregivers and those with dementia face so that they feel they can speak more openly. Give those who are impacted by dementia an opportunity to connect with one another. Consider flexible or modified work arrangements. Explore employee-assistance programs. Train managers to notice the signs of dementia and be attuned to caregiver stress. Put employee caregiver policies in place and ensure that employees know they will be treated with care upon disclosing a diagnosis. Ask a dementia society for examples of solid employment policies for caregivers and people with dementia. Good policies will help attract and retain faithful staff.

Encourage businesses to put practices and policies in place

Businesses can help people with dementia and their caregivers feel like they are a part of their community. Consider identifying a dementia champion in the workplace. Training staff to be dementia-friendly can help them become more sensitive. Connect with a dementia society that offers practical tips: for example, on how to respond compassionately if someone forgets their PIN number, or has difficulty counting money, or is agitated. Becoming dementia-friendly doesn't necessarily come with a heavy price tag. Simple modifications can help. Clear signage at entrances and exits and advising staff to proactively offer help if someone appears lost or confused can help. In fact, accommodating the needs of people with dementia can be good for business. In one study, 83 percent of people with memory problems switched their shopping habits to places that were more accessible.[65] Offering dementia-friendly hours during the week – during which the volume of music is lowered, lights are dimmed the lights, and announcements kept to a minimum – can draw those with dementia back to your business. Contact your local dementia or Alzheimer's Society for tips about how your business cannot just help but benefit from becoming more welcoming.

Plan dementia-friendly public spaces

How we organize ourselves and design our living environments either widen or limit our circles of care. The majority of people with dementia live at home, either alone or with a caregiver.[66] If public spaces are not designed to include them, then they are confined to their home. Widening circles of care means advocating for public spaces that are inclusive. All development and public space planning should ensure that everyone can access services and opportunities, and specifically take into account the needs of people with dementia, including how they navigate outside the home. Researchers Lynne Mitchell and Elizabeth Burton identify six factors that make neighbourhoods more accessible to those with dementia: familiarity, legibility, distinctiveness, accessibility, comfort, and safety. Practically, Mitchell and Burton recommend clear sidewalks, access to less-busy routes, and wide pathways for ease of movement. Because people with dementia are more likely to use landmarks than maps to find their way, planting unique trees or scented plants at juncture points and ensuring that they are clearly marked can reduce stress and help people find their way.[67]

Act as active advocates and challenge stigma

"They don't think I know what's going on," Gerry told me one day. "As soon as I got this damned dementia, the neighbours assumed I was incompetent. They hardly look at me."

People like Gerry are routinely stigmatized. The Alzheimer Society's *Canadian Charter of Rights for People with Dementia*[68] states that people have the right to be free from discrimination of any kind. All of us have a responsibility to uphold the charter by becoming advocates. Sometimes it means gently challenging family and friends who talk about people who have dementia as "empty shells." Other times, it can look like shifting the decision-making about care to the person with dementia, or like suggesting that people with dementia participate on decision-making boards. Be aware that challenges people with dementia face can be laced with other systems of oppression. For people over the age of 65, for example, discrimination can be compounded by ageism. Those who belong to culturally marginalized communities can face even more significant barriers when it comes to accessing support. Intentionally bring together those with dementia (especially those on the margins) and community leaders for public consultations. Life-enhancing ideas surface when we truly listen to one another.

SCRIPTURE: LUKE 5:27–32

After this he went out and saw a tax collector named Levi, sitting at the tax booth; and he said to him, "Follow me." And he got up, left everything, and followed him. Then Levi gave a great banquet for him in his house; and there was a large crowd of tax collectors and others sitting at the table with them. The Pharisees and their scribes were complaining to his disciples, saying, "Why do you eat and drink with tax collectors and sinners?" Jesus answered, "Those who are well have no need of a physician, but those who are sick; I have come to call not the righteous but sinners to repentance."

QUESTIONS FOR REFLECTION AND DISCUSSION

1. Name three ways that your community could better support your caregiving work.
2. How could the physical environments you find yourself in be more conducive to caregiving?
3. If you could change one thing to make society more dementia friendly, what would it be?
4. How did Jesus widen circles of compassion through his care?

SPIRITUAL PRACTICE: SAYING GRACE

Jesus and the apostle Paul routinely said grace, a type of thanksgiving prayer shared before meals. The word "grace" comes from the Latin *gratia*, meaning thanks. Grace literally means saying thank you. Although, it's by no means a new spiritual practice, grace continues to be countercultural. It's an admission that we are not wholly independent but rely on God and on others for the gift of nourishment. Expand grace to a mealtime spiritual practice of gratitude.

1. Before your meal, pause to be grateful. Say your favourite grace or try a new one.
2. Be mindful as you are eating, conscious of your food and where it came from. Give thanks for the growers, producers, and all the elements of nature for the blessing of food that is before you. Name as many as you can. Hold them in prayer.
3. Take time to savour what you are eating and drinking. Don't rush. Feel the food in your mouth. Truly experience the pleasure of taste. Give thanks for the enjoyment.

4. Consider those who do not have the abundance of food you have. Hold them in prayer. Similarly, reflect on those who cannot approach the tables of power in our society. Hold them in prayer, too.

5. Visualize the food and drink entering your body and refreshing you, energizing you to care with compassion.

6. Pause to be grateful when you are finished.

PRAYER

Thank you for Jesus' witness at the table, O God.

There, he showed me how to widen the circles of my care.

There, he befriended sinners, performed miracles, and established sacraments.

There, he taught important lessons about humility, community, and friendship.

There, he prayed for just what he needed, no more and no less – daily bread.

Here and now, O God, set the tables of my life with Jesus' values.

Here and now, let his care multiply.

Let me pass it out like fresh bread,

a sustaining comfort,

a source of hope

broken open,

shared

with anyone hungry for love.

Amen.

12

Feeling Grief and Finding Hope

"I do half of my stuff to keep [her] happy.
I go to programs for her. I have a personal
support worker for her. Love is a two-way street.
I'm thinking of her very much."
– Dennis

Picture a storm. The most wicked of storms. Hear the sound of the thunder. See the slash of the lighting. Feel the rain beating down. You are in a boat at sea, feeling the waves rise and roll beneath you. You are terrified. You've never felt more out of control. It's an effort just to stay on the boat. To hang on and in.

That's how Ruth described how her days caring for her husband who was in the late stages of dementia felt. "It's like being in a boat in the middle of the sea," she said. "Sometimes I don't know from one minute to the next whether I'm going to capsize."

It had been four years since the official diagnosis; Ruth said she felt that way from the beginning. Like something alien had taken over their lives. She resented the illness. In truth, she didn't want to be a caregiver and felt guilty and selfish for saying that she was sad about the ways it derailed her life, their life together.

Dementia doesn't just happen to the person who has received the diagnosis, it happens to everyone who loves them, too. Often, illness interrupts life as we know it. Plans go by the wayside. Life changes colour. Whether we want to or not, dementia forces us to admit vulnerability. It draws hard feelings to the surface: fear, shame, guilt, anger, and sadness. Sometimes, the feelings swell and threaten to overtake us.

So what do you do with those feelings, the heavy ones you feel ashamed to have or conflicted about? Especially the feeling of grief and loss?

When we care for people with dementia, we know that they aren't going to get better. There will be good days and bad days, but ultimately there is no cure. There is no way around the hard reality. It can be excruciatingly painful to care for someone who isn't going to get better. In these instances, our care can be laced with grief.

From experience, we know we can face many losses in the course of a long illness: the loss of role, intimacy, financial stability, home ... Sometimes those losses can feel overwhelming, the grief palpable.

While most of us are familiar with grief that happens after death, "anticipatory grief" or the loss we feel before a person dies is less well known. Anticipatory grief is particularly difficult to express because it leaves us hanging between life and death, losing while alive but not yet being able to grieve the final loss that is death.[69]

I can't count how many people have told me that anticipatory grief feels worse than grief after death, partly because it feels unnatural to grieve a person while they are still present and it's taboo to talk about it. But anticipatory grief is real and natural. It's also okay to feel relief when our loved one has died, regardless of the circumstances that led to their death.

It's often said that grief is the flip side of love. We grieve most for those we love most, or for those we most long for. Our grief stems from our deepest blessing. Intuitively, we know that. But knowing we have loved and continue to love doesn't make grief easier to deal with.

Feelings are not good or bad in and of themselves. They are neutral. Anger itself, for example, isn't wrong, but the way we channel anger can be. There is no wrong or right way to feel. Instead of passing judgment on yourself for feeling the way you do, congratulate yourself for naming your feelings. Seriously. Give yourself a gold star for knowing how you feel. If you can begin to articulate why you feel that way, that's even better.

Our hardest feelings feel heavier when we carry them alone. Sometimes, we hide our feelings from the person we are caring for to shield them. And sometimes we hide our feelings from family and friends so as not to burden them, or because we fear what they will think of us if we disclose what's on our heart. If that's the case for you, consider seeking out a non-judgmental confidant who you feel you can be honest with, whether that is a friend, therapist, religious leader, or support group.

Know that whatever you are feeling, you are in good company.

When Ruth shared her hard feelings with me and what it was like to be sloshed about in the boat, I told her that her experience reminded me of the story in Matthew's gospel where Jesus is in the boat with his disciples and they are freaking out in the midst of a massive storm (Matthew 8:23–27).

What was Jesus doing? Sleeping. Sawing logs! I don't know about you, but when a storm threatens my life, the last thing I can do is wind down enough to drift off.

The story continues that the disciples wake Jesus up and the first question out of his lips is "Why are you afraid?" What a stupid question! There are any number of obvious things to be afraid of: never getting back to shore, not being able to bail fast enough, getting thrown overboard, being struck by lightning ... Yet Jesus seems to be telling his disciples that they need to be less afraid because he is there. And in a head spinning moment, he stands up, tells the storm to stop, and, miraculously, it does.

I sometimes wish there was an off button for my hardest feelings, but I know that denying them or ignoring them doesn't make me feel any better. In fact, it tends to make things worse. When the feelings pile up, I don't sleep. I get grouchy. I feel depressed. I either eat too much or not enough.

There were a lot of feelings in Jesus' boat: anxiety, panic, doom, despair. Yet Jesus himself represented other feelings – peacefulness, hope, calm – and herein lies the message. Yes, hard feelings accompany many of the storms we find ourselves in, but there are other feelings, too. Ones we too often don't seek out, fail to see, or ignore. These are the ones that help us sleep at night, focus on possibilities, and energize us with hope.

To repeat, there's no denying the hard feelings. They are there. And it's okay and right that they are. It's just that they aren't the *only* feelings we have. They are always on board, but we shouldn't necessarily let them run the ship.

When do you feel calm in the midst of a "storm"? Throughout your day, when are you most at ease? When does your fear slip away? These moments and whatever contributes to them are cause for gratitude. Increasingly, researchers are finding that practicing gratitude is an antidote to stress and anxiety. By no stretch am I saying that we should be grateful for illness, but despite illness there are blessings we can be thankful for.

HaKarat HaTov is the Hebrew expression for gratitude.[70] It means "recognizing the good." Not the good that *might* arrive in the future, but the good that *already* exists in the now. Noting what you are grateful for during the day can give positive, thankful thoughts a chance to take the wheel.

When we are extremely fearful, we tend to micro-focus on what we are afraid of. Makes sense, right? After all, it's the scary thing we need to confront. But in the face of something that feels larger than life, we can become stuck and feel like the outcome is out of our hands.

It's true that there is no cure for dementia, but that doesn't mean we have no control over our lives. You may not be able to control the storm, but the boat is yours to navigate. Name some things about your experience that you can control. Keep expanding the list. "I am only one, but still I am one; I cannot do everything, but still I can do something; and just because I cannot do everything, I will not refuse to do the something that I can do," wrote Jeanie Ashley Bates Greenough at the turn of the 20th century.[71]

Moisture and instability are the two key ingredients in a massive storm. There's not much any one of us can do to control either. We may well resent the moisture, the instability, and the storm itself, but wasting energy while we are in the boat by resenting the things we can't control isn't going to help. Storms do what they do. We would do better to accept the storm than fight the reality of it. As caregivers, strength comes from adaptability.

The idea of "going with the flow" is widely attributed to the second-century Roman Emperor Marcus Aurelius, who frequently ruminated on life's transitions. "Time is a sort of river of passing events, and strong is its current; no sooner is a thing brought to sight than it is swept by and another takes its place, and this too will be swept away," he writes. In his writings, Aurelius was coming to terms with the fact that change is inevitable. "Going with the flow" is a way of capturing the idea of being adaptable.

I don't know about you, but when I wake up in the morning, I already have in mind a vision of a perfect day. Even if the day I have planned isn't going to be exciting, I still have a picture of what would make it good. I have a set of expectations: my computer is going to start, I will be able to attend to errands with ease, my coworkers are going to be decent. When events fail to live up to my expectations, I don't go with the flow as easily. Admittedly, I don't have the most flexible of mindsets.

After inhaling my coffee and making the bed, the first thing I do every morning is make a "to do" list for the day. I want so badly to make my days "count" that I am very stuck on checking things off my list. When things take longer than I had planned, or worse, when events derail my list, I can get flustered.

A couple of months ago, I had invited five family members over for dinner. Two said they couldn't make it so I planned for three. An hour before dinner, the pair called to let me know they were coming after all. My first thought wasn't "that's great" – although I was gracious enough to say I was glad. On the inside, I launched into panic mode. When I rummaged around the freezer and couldn't find anything suitable, I grew agitated. I was annoyed at the lack of consideration. I snapped at my brother who was visiting: "Don't they know that I need a bit of warning?"

I have a vision of my role as the matriarch in the family. I have always been the provider and expressed love with food. I wasn't upset with my family because they were dropping in. In fact, I love it when they do. But on that day when I didn't have enough food, what I was *really* upset about was not being able to live up to my own expectations of myself. What kind of provider am I if I can't provide?

To-do lists can keep us focused. And the roles we assume in life can provide meaning. But both can also lend to inflexible expectations. That means when the storms come – and they *will* come because that's what they do – we may not be as adaptable and resilient as we need to be.

Learning when to let go and go with the flow are critical skills for caregivers. Dementia can lead to unpredictable moments. Adopting a flexible mindset and living in the moment means focusing on what we *do* have rather than on what we don't have, on what is and can still go right rather than on what is wrong, and adjusting our expectations of ourselves.

Abandon perfect. There is no such thing as a perfect day, a perfect life, or a perfect world. On the whole, expecting that everything will unfold as it should or resenting that it hasn't done so will inevitably lead to despair. Instead, seek out and dwell on moments of beauty. They are everywhere.

I was invited into one such beautiful moment when I interviewed a couple about their experience of dementia as I wrote this book. Here is a verbatim excerpt.

Me: Donna, I've heard you say that dementia is not the end and in fact that it can be fun. What's fun about it?

Donna: We get around more. It's wonderful. We say to each other, "We have to." We do social activities. We try to do something every day. Dennis is involved with programs with the Alzheimer's society. It's about connecting so that you have a support group and can socialize. Dennis gets out every day to a program. Yesterday, a personal support worker started. She came to our home. She just hung out with Dennis and they got to know each other. We are trying to take advantage of the wealth of support available to us.

Dennis: We try to keep positive and keep going ... dragged, and crawl into bed and pull the covers over my head. That's a problem right there. The dementia has affected the ability to pull up words. Thought process. Can't verbalize. That's frustrating.

Donna: You have to take each day as it comes. If you think too much about the past, you can get sad. If you think too much about the future, you can become anxious. So we think about today and have fun. Today we are hanging a wreath outside and going grocery shopping.

Dennis: I do half of my stuff to keep you happy. I go to programs for her. I have a personal support worker for her. Love is a two-way street. I'm thinking of her very much.

Donna teared up as Dennis expressed what he did for her, how he went along to make her happy, how much he thought about her. There it was: love. Clear, transparent love in all its finest reciprocity.

Love is present. We have to look for it differently, though. We may not hear it through the usual conventions. We may sense it in a touch. In hanging a wreath. In togetherness. Once we expand our view of how love is mediated to us, we begin to see it anew. We experience joy.

Silver linings and rainbows aren't wishful thinking. They are reality. We are surrounded in love and blessing. We are blessed to be a blessing. Beauty and blessing are the wellspring of hope. Where do you find beauty and blessing in your day? Do you see it in yourself?

Dementia affects us but it doesn't *define* us. It doesn't define us as people who are diagnosed or as caregivers. *Love* defines us. It is the essence of who we are created to be. When we are most loving, we are most holy.

"For I am convinced that neither death, nor life, nor angels, nor rulers, nor things present, nor things to come, nor powers, nor height, nor depth, nor anything else in all creation, will be able to separate us from the love of God," writes Paul in the book of Romans (Romans 8:38–39). That's because love is all around us and it shines through us. Love isn't contingent on memory or in a brain that functions normally. It's constant. Present in every storm.

Caring can be hard. It can be laced with guilt and grief. And it can be filled with beauty and hope. Coming to a place of acceptance, seeking beauty, expressing gratitude, sharing our hardest feelings, letting go of what we can't control and focusing on what we can control, giving up on the idea of perfection, adjusting our expectations, affirming ourselves and staying grounded in the spirit of love can all steer us in the direction of hope on our most desperate days.

Know that your care is blessed, no matter how hard or fraught with conflicted feelings. Caregiving is meaningful and noble. A holy calling. As a witness, companion, healer, and advocate, you transform lives. To someone, you mean the world. Not everyone can say that.

In case you don't hear this enough: Thank you.

SCRIPTURE: MATTHEW 8:23–27

And when he got into the boat, his disciples followed him. A windstorm arose on the sea, so great that the boat was being swamped by the waves; but he was asleep. And they went and woke him up, saying, "Lord, save us! We are perishing!" And he said to them, "Why are you afraid, you of little faith?" Then he got up and rebuked the winds and the sea; and there was a dead calm. They were amazed, saying, "What sort of man is this, that even the winds and the sea obey him?"

QUESTIONS FOR REFLECTION AND DISCUSSION

1. What are your hardest feelings? What makes them hard? What frightens you most?
2. Where do you experience hope?
3. Jesus epitomizes calm in Matthew's story. When are you most calm?

4. Looking back, when in your life has God/the presence of divine love calmed a storm?

SPIRITUAL PRACTICE: THE EXAMEN

St. Ignatius of Loyola included a prayer called the "Examen" in his *Spiritual Exercises*. The name "Examen" comes from the Latin word for examination and is a way of reviewing the day through a spiritual lens. There are various versions of the Examen, but here are six steps typically found in each.

1. Notice God's presence. Say a prayer of thanks for God's love.
2. Pray for wisdom to understand how God is active throughout your day.
3. Reflect on your day from the very beginning when you woke up until now. What did you do? How did you feel?
4. What thoughts ran through your mind in each of these moments and what did you say or do?
5. Consider when you drew nearer to God in these moments and when you drew further away.
6. Ask for God's grace on your day tomorrow, identifying specific moments when you anticipate needing to sense God's love.

PRAYER

Hold my hardest feelings, Holy One.

Hold them because they are too heavy for me to carry.

Hold them so that they don't hold me down.

And as you hold them, hold me, too.

Hold me close to your eternal and infinite heart.

Whisper to me there

a word of peace,

a word of courage,

a word of grace,

a word of hope.

Amen.

NOTES

1. "avodah," *The Jewish Language Project*, https://jel.jewish-languages.org/words/1863

2. "Dementia," *World Health Organization*, https://tinyurl.com/znantmnm

3. "What Is Alzheimer's Disease?" *Alzheimer's Association*, https://tinyurl.com/3zthx8st

4. Jesse F. Ballenger, "Framing Confusion: Dementia, Society and History," *AMA Journal of Ethics*. 2017; 19(7):713-719, https://tinyurl.com/295476sw

5. Ibid.

6. Elizabeth Liebert, "Discernment for Our Times. A Practice with Postmodern Implications," *Studies in Spirituality* (2008), 18:333–355.

7. "Caregiver Identity Discrepancy and Implications for Practice," *YouTube*, https://tinyurl.com/h826csx7

8. "I Live with Dementia: Ken and Mark," *Alzheimer Society of Canada*, https://ilivewithdementia.ca/ken-and-mark/

9. "Implicit Biases and People with Disabilities," *American Bar Association*, January 7, 2019, https://tinyurl.com/xnyd62ca

10. "Some Issues in Locke's Philosophy of Mind," *Stanford Encyclopedia of Philosophy*, https://tinyurl.com/k84fkhkz

11. Kristine N. Williams et al., "Elderspeak Communication: Impact on Dementia Care," *PMC (PubMed Central)*, https://tinyurl.com/e8vpc9zw – See also Steve Balsis and Brian D. Carpenter, "Evaluations of Elderspeak in a Caregiving Contest," Research Gate, https://tinyurl.com/ytr3ujwc – and Ruth E. Herman and Kristine N. Williams, "Elderspeak's Influence on Resistiveness to Care: Behavioral Events," *PMC (PubMed Central)*, https://tinyurl.com/kcbhvn9j

12. Siva Banovic, Lejla Junuzovic Zunic, and Osam Sinanovic, "Communication Difficulties as a Result of Dementia," *PMC (PubMed Central)*, https://tinyurl.com/uc2weszc

13. Alan and Barbara Pease, *The Definitive Book of Body Language*, chapter 1 accessed at https://tinyurl.com/2ukp9zc9

14. "Late Stages: Communication and Activities," *Alzheimer's Research and Resource Foundation*, https://tinyurl.com/dzashvb9

15. Nathan M. D'Cunha et al., "Psychological Responses in People Living with Dementia after an Art Gallery Intervention," *IOS Press Content Library*, https://tinyurl.com/rebszvts

16. Corita Kent and Jan Steward, *Learning by Heart: Teachings to Free the Creative Spirit* (New York: Skyhorse Publishing, 2008), 28.

17. TimeSlips, https://www.timeslips.org/

18. Abigail Fagan, "How the Arts Can Reshape Dementia Care: Anne Basting explains how to connect to people with dementia," *Psychology Today*, https://tinyurl.com/tzva2vbu

19. Alzheimer Poetry Project, http://www.alzpoetry.com

20. Songwriting Works, https://songwritingworks.org/

21. Opening Minds through Art, https://www.scrippsoma.org/about/

22. Michael Glover, "Late flowering or failing: Did work by artists like De Kooning, Renoir, Matisse and Monet decline in old age?" *Independent*, October 15, 2017, https://tinyurl.com/p4ytkpy5

23. John Whitfield, "Brain disease shaped Boléro," *Nature*, January 22, 2002, https://tinyurl.com/au36jkun

24. Thomas Merton, *No Man Is an Island* (Shambhala Publications, 2005).

25. "Tallest Man Ever," *Guinness World Records*, https://tinyurl.com/4axda437

26. "Managing Behaviour Changes," *Alzheimer's Society of Calgary*, https://tinyurl.com/t8usj3se

27. "Medications and Dementia," University of California San Francisco (UCSF), https://tinyurl.com/2bh2thsd

28. "Wandering: Who's at Risk?" *Alzheimer's Association*, https://tinyurl.com/4pufm24z

29. "Walking About," *Alzheimer's Society*, https://tinyurl.com/re26n6mj

30. "Wandering and Alzheimer's Disease," *National Institute of Aging*, https://tinyurl.com/rdsupt66

31. "Ways to Prevent Wandering," *WebMD*, https://tinyurl.com/2zwpta9a

32. "'I want to go home: What to say to someone in care with dementia," *Alzheimer's Society*, https://tinyurl.com/4h7xtzw6

33. "3 Ways to Respond When Someone with Alzheimer's Says I Want to Go Home," *DailyCaring*, https://tinyurl.com/kcss54kx

34. "Kind Ways to Respond When a Person with Dementia Forgets Someone Has Died," *Women's Alzheimer's Movement*, https://tinyurl.com/jtzw9t3t

35. "Driving Information and Contract," *Alzheimer's Association*, https://tinyurl.com/cc29m36p

36. "Driving with Dementia," *Alzheimer's Society*, https://tinyurl.com/4jvuenz5

37. "Treatment of Inappropriate Behavior in Dementia," *PubMed Central*, https://tinyurl.com/z84m3dzj

38. "Caring for the Elderly: Dealing with Resistance," *Mayo Clinic*, https://tinyurl.com/4vztr5t2

39. "Suspicions and Delusions," *Alzheimer's Association*, https://tinyurl.com/bmd3ypav

40. "Caregiver Stress Check," *Alzheimer's Association*, https://tinyurl.com/jrxnkw7e See also "Caregiver Stress," *Alzheimer's Association*, https://tinyurl.com/uwzxfhsc

41. "The Radical History of Self-Care," *BBC Radio Four*, https://tinyurl.com/6jp9yy5a

42. "Understanding Caregiver Burnout: Symptoms, Treatment & Prevention," *Care Squared*, https://caresquared.com.au/caregiver-burnout/

43. "The Experiences and Needs of Older Caregivers in Canada," *Statistics Canada*, https://tinyurl.com/2xjkrz4w

44. "Caregivers," *Anxiety & Depression Association of America*, https://tinyurl.com/3wf2eh3d

45. Rachel Naomi Remen, *Kitchen Table Wisdom: Stories That Heal* (New York: Penguin, 1996).

46. Stephen R. Covey, *The 7 Habits of Highly Effective People* (New York: Simon & Schuster, 1989).

47. Arthur Frank, "Illness and Narrative" (Keynote speech, Department of Sociology, University of Calgary), https://tinyurl.com/4kxhnrrd

48. Eric Cassell, "The Nature of Suffering and the Goals of Medicine," *Artbeat,* October 12, 2014, https://tinyurl.com/2wak7k4b

49. "Explaining Dementia to Children and Young People," *Alzheimer's Society,* https://tinyurl.com/3f3ucvav

50. "How to Talk to Children about the Serious Illness of a Loved One," *Harvard Health Blog*; entry by Dr. Claire McCarthy, December 2019, https://tinyurl.com/sch78cuw

51. "Just for Kids," *Alzheimer Society of Canada,* https://tinyurl.com/ysmez6vh

52. *Alzheimer's Research UK: Dementia Explained,* https://tinyurl.com/9pshr7aj

53. *Dementia in My Family,* https://dementiainmyfamily.org.au/

54. *The Dragon Story, YouTube,* https://tinyurl.com/6r9mxfs

55. "Parent's Guide: Helping Children and Teens Understand Alzheimer's Disease," *Alzheimer's Association,* https://tinyurl.com/fmcrbs4x

56. "Dementia Resource Suite for Schools: Creating a Dementia-Friendly Generation," *Alzheimer's Society,* https://tinyurl.com/bemwm22r

57. "Dan's Story," *Alzheimer's Research UK: Dementia Explained,* https://tinyurl.com/wsn3hu2

58. Robert J. Karris, *Eating Your Way through Luke's Gospel* (Collegeville, Minnesota: Order of Saint Benedict, 2006), 97.

59. Albert Einstein, *Good Reads,* https://tinyurl.com/36kzeez5

60. "The Secret of Happiness? Here's Some Advice from the Longest-running Study on Happiness," *Harvard Health Blog,* entry by Matthew Solan, October 5, 2017, https://tinyurl.com/557vwhuf

61. "Social Isolation and Loneliness in Older Adults: Opportunities for the Health Care System," *NCBI (National Center for Biotechology Information),* https://tinyurl.com/44s9t542

62. "World's Largest Dementia Study Reveals Lack of Understanding about the Condition," *London School of Economics and Political Science,* September 20, 2019, https://tinyurl.com/432jjet8

63. *Silver Alert Canada,* https://silveralertcanada.ca/

64. "Building Dementia-friendly Communities: A Priority for Everyone," *Alzheimer's Society,* https://tinyurl.com/ufr7w6pd, 7

65. "Building Dementia Friendly Organizations," *CLH Health Care*, January 13, 2020, https://tinyurl.com/4a9kkc3j

66. "Dementia in Home and Community Care," *Canadian Institute for Health Information*, https://tinyurl.com/4a7bdzah

67. Lynne Mitchell and Elizabeth Burton, "Designing Dementia-Friendly Neighbour-hoods: Helping People with Dementia to Get Out and About," *Journal of Integrated Care*, November 2010, https://tinyurl.com/2swtcxa9

68. "The Canadian Charter of Rights for People with Dementia," *Alzheimer Society of Canada*, https://tinyurl.com/47hvwfjv

69. Trevor Josephson, "Ambiguous and Anticipatory Grief" (presentation, Parkinson Society British Columbia, March 25, 2020), https://tinyurl.com/2pk37nkp

70. "*HaKarat HaTov*: Jewish Thanksgiving and Jewish Living," *Congregation Rodeph Shalom: Blog*, https://tinyurl.com/nx5z4t3d

71. Jeanie Ashley Bates Greenough, *A Year of Beautiful Thoughts* (New York, NY: Thomas Y. Crowell & Co.,1902), n172. https://archive.org/details/yearofbeautifult001150mbp/page/n172/mode/2up

THE AUTHOR

As an ordained minister, Trisha Elliott has supported caregivers of people with dementia for over 20 years and was honoured to receive the Queens Theological College alumni achievement award for ministry excellence. As a writer, cultural creative, and artist, Trisha has won numerous national and international awards 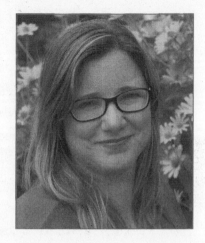 for features in a variety of genres. She has contributed to a handful of books and was a guest religion commentator at the National Arts Centre. Trisha lives in Ottawa, Canada, where she has only moderate success coaxing her two teenage sons to explore forests and largely fails to convince them to eat anything she has foraged. Visit her online at trishaelliott.com.

THE ARCHITECTURE OF HOPE
Douglas MacLeod

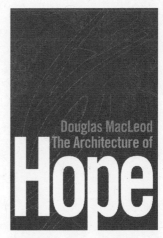

Architect and educator Douglas MacLeod offers a stark and immediately compelling glimpse into the future, 15 years hence, in which we can live and work together to build better communities for tomorrow.

This insightful and compelling book imagines the idea of cooperative communities where people can produce more energy than they use; purify more water than they pollute; grow more food than they consume; and recycle more waste than they produce, with technologies that already exist or that will be within our grasp in a few years.

Most important of all, the people of the community own and profit from these resources.

The Architecture of Hope depicts a way of living that is decentralized, re-localized, and regenerative. And possible.

ISBN 978-1-77343-174-1

80 pages, 4.75" x 7" paperback, $12.95

THE VOICE OF THE GALILEAN

The story of a life, a journey,
a discovery, a gift, and a fate

Rex Weyler

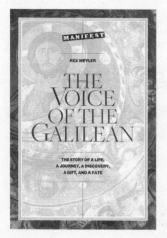

Rex Weyler's *The Voice of the Galilean* stands as one of the most clear, compelling, and concise tellings of the life and teachings of Jesus ever written. Excerpted and updated from his seminal book *The Jesus Sayings: The Quest for His Authentic Message* – a brilliant synthesis of the work of international Bible scholars and some 200 ancient sources, including the gospels of Thomas and Mary – *The Voice of the Galilean* distills the teachings of Jesus with crystal clarity, sensitivity, insight, and passion. Equally important, Weyler challenges readers to bear "witness" to Jesus' message today, in their own lives.

ISBN 978-1-77343-155-0

96 pages, 4.25" x 6.25" paperback, $12.95

FOR EVERYTHING A SEASON

The Wisdom of Traditional Values
in Turbulent Times

Warren Johnson

For Everything a Season reignites the sacred flame. Warren Johnson urges us to recommit to faith, while maintaining our reason. Guided by traditional principles embedded in the great teachings of the New and Old Testaments, he offers a hopeful path to creating a modern ecosystem where every individual consumes and creates in balance with the sacred whole. In this way, we do away 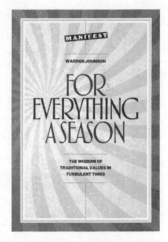 with excess, make reparations for our past, and ultimately lead a happier, healthier life.

ISBN 978-1-77343-166-6
96 pages, 4.25" x 6.25" paperback, $12.95

WOOD LAKE

Imagining, living, and telling
the faith story.

WOOD LAKE IS THE FAITH STORY COMPANY.

It has told

- the story of the seasons of the earth, the people of God, and the place and purpose of faith in the world;
- the story of the faith journey, from birth to death;
- the story of Jesus and the churches that carry his message.

Wood Lake has been telling stories for more than 35 years. During that time, it has given form and substance to the words, songs, pictures, and ideas of hundreds of storytellers.

Those stories have taken a multitude of forms – parables, poems, drawings, prayers, epiphanies, songs, books, paintings, hymns, curricula – all driven by a common mission of serving those on the faith journey.

WOOD LAKE PUBLISHING INC.

485 Beaver Lake Road, Kelowna, BC, CanadaV4V 1S5

250.766.2778

www.woodlake.com